'With humility and uncanny insight, Arno Geiger shines
a pure and natural light upon a subject we too often shy
away from, turning it into something very positive and
uplifting. This book is a gift to all of us who struggle
with life and death and all its jagged edges.'

Ray Mattinson, Blackwell, Oxford

'A moving and revealing depiction of the reality of
dementia. Told tenderly with love and respect, it is a
celebration of humanity in difficult times and a testament
to the importance of understanding one another.'

Claire Grint, Cogito Books, Hexham

'A deeply affecting examination of the hope to be found amidst
illness and loss. Geiger writes with clear eyes and an open heart.'

Marion Rankine, Foyles Charing Cross, London

'Geiger writes about family, old age and illness with elegant
poignancy and the kind of wisdom that only comes from
painful experience, but there is strength and hope here too.
This is writing that warms your heart even as it breaks it.'

Jenny Buckland, Heywood Hill bookshop, London

'I loved everything about *The Old King in His Exile* and read it in one sitting. A really moving (both sad and joyous) treat.'

'A love letter from a son to his father, *The Old King in His Exile* completely avoids sentimentalism, yet is never lacking in humour and compassion. It made me realise that the sum of a life is the whole life and not just its ending.'

'Arno Geiger invites us to share in precious time spent with his father and it feels like an honour to do so. Always honest about the brutal realities of dementia, Geiger nevertheless looks for the man and not the illness. With prose so beautifully simple yet striking it begs you to read passages aloud, I doubt there is anybody who could read this book and not be deeply moved.'

'This book is startlingly unsentimental, and yet a painful and touchingly realised picture of dementia, and the way it alters relationships between the sufferer and the people closest to them. It is incredibly relatable and emotionally provocative, but it also becomes a more general meditation on life and the continuous process of ageing.'

THE OLD KING IN HIS EXILE

Arno Geiger

Translated by
Stefan Tobler

SHEFFIELD

First published in English translation in 2017 by And Other Stories
www.andotherstories.org

9 8 7 6 5 4 3 2 1

ISBN: 978-1-908276-88-9
eBook ISBN: 978-1-908276-89-6

Typesetter: Tetragon, London; Proofreader: Sarah Terry; Typefaces: Linotype Swift Neue and Verlag; Cover Design: Edward Bettison; Cover Illustration: Aurelia Lange; Printed and bound by the CPI Group (UK) Ltd, Croydon, CR0 4YY.

A catalogue record for this book is available from the British Library.

And Other Stories is supported by public funding from Arts Council England.

The translation of this work was supported by a grant from the Goethe-Institut, which is funded by the German Ministry of Foreign Affairs, and by the Austrian Federal Chancellery.

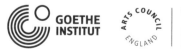

Supported using public funding by
**ARTS COUNCIL
ENGLAND**

THE OLD KING
IN HIS EXILE

You have to show what is most universal
In a personal way.

HOKUSAI

When I was six, my grandfather stopped recognising me. He lived in the house down the hill from ours, and because I cut through his orchard on the way to school, occasionally he threw a piece of wood at me, saying I had no business on his land. Sometimes, though, he liked to see me and would come over, calling me Helmut. That didn't mean anything to me either. My grandfather died. I forgot what had happened – until the illness started in my father.

In Russia there's a saying that nothing in life returns except our mistakes. And that they become worse in our old age. As my father had always been somewhat eccentric, we told ourselves that the slip-ups he started to make after his retirement were because he allowed himself to lose interest in his surroundings. It seemed typical of him. So for years we nagged, urging him to pull himself together.

Now I'm seized by a silent rage at all that wasted effort, because we were scolding the person instead of the disease. 'Please, don't let yourself go!' we said a hundred times, and our father put up with us patiently, as if believing things are easiest if you resign yourself to them in good time. He didn't want to resist his forgetfulness and never used any memory aids. That way, he couldn't mistakenly think someone else had put a knot in his handkerchief as a reminder. Nor did he fight tooth and nail against his mental decline, and he didn't once try to broach the subject, although – with hindsight – he must have known it was serious by the mid-nineties at the latest. If he had said to one of his children, 'I'm sorry, my brain is letting me down,' everyone would have been able to deal with the situation better. As it was, for years there was a cat-and-mouse game where our father was a mouse, we were mice, and the disease was the cat.

That first nerve-wracking phase, marked by uncertainties and insecurities, is behind us. Although I still don't like to think about it, I now understand that there's a difference between giving up because you don't want to try and giving up because you know you're beaten. Our father accepted that he was beaten. Having arrived at that stage of life where his mental powers were on the wane, he staked everything on maintaining inner composure. Which, in the absence of effective medication, is also a practical solution for relatives who have to deal with this wretched illness.

In *The Curtain*, Milan Kundera writes: 'Faced with the unavoidable defeat we call life, the only thing left to us is the attempt to understand it.'

I imagine dementia's intermediate phase, the phase my father is in, more or less like this: you're wrenched out of your sleep, you don't know where you are, everything whirls around you – countries, years, people. You try to get your bearings, but you can't. Everything continues to spin – the dead, the living, memories, dreamlike hallucinations, snatches of sentences that don't mean anything to you – and this condition doesn't change for the rest of the day.

*

When I'm back home in Wolfurt, as I am only occasionally, since a number of us share the burden of care, I wake my father around nine. He lies under his blanket, in shock, but he's accustomed enough to people he doesn't know stepping into his bedroom that he doesn't complain.

'Wouldn't you like to get up?' I ask him in a friendly voice. And to inject a little optimism, I add, 'What a wonderful life we have.'

Sceptical, he struggles to his feet. 'You, perhaps,' he says.

I pass him his socks. He looks at the socks for a while with raised eyebrows and then asks, 'Where's the third one?'

I help him with dressing, to speed it up. He is willing to let me do it. Then I guide him down to the kitchen for breakfast. Afterwards I ask him to go and shave. He says, with a wink, 'I'd have been better off staying at home. I won't be visiting you again in a hurry.'

I show him the way to the toilet. He sings, 'Oh dear, oh dear . . . oh dear, oh dear,' playing for time.

'If you shave, you'll look sharp,' I say.

He follows hesitantly. 'If you say so,' he murmurs. Looking in the mirror, he puts his hands on the hair sticking up on his head, pressing hard so that the hair actually stays down. He looks at himself again, declares, 'Almost like new!' and thanks me warmly with a smile.

He has started thanking me a lot. A few days ago, without any obvious reason, he said, 'I thank you most kindly in advance.'

I respond encouragingly to such utterances now. 'You're welcome,' I say, or 'Don't mention it,' or 'Happy to help.' In my experience affirmative answers, which give my father the feeling that everything is fine, are better than the probing questions I used to ask, which only embarrassed and unsettled him. None of us like to answer questions that, if understood at all, only make us aware of our own inadequacies.

At first, the process of adjusting was painful and draining. Parents seem, to their children, strong and able to stand up to life's unpleasant surprises, so we children are much harder on our parents for their increasingly visible weaknesses than we would be on other people. But over time I have settled into the new role pretty well. And I have learnt that you measure the life of someone affected by dementia differently.

If my father wants to say thank you, let him say thank you, even if there's no obvious reason, and if he wants to complain, let him complain, whether or not his judgement is corroborated by the world of facts. He has no world beyond his dementia. As part of his family, I can only hope to remove some of the situation's bitterness by allowing a sick man his muddled reality.

As my father can no longer cross the bridge into my world, I have to go over to his. There, within the limits of his own mental state, beyond the wider society based on objectivity and linear goals, he is still an impressive man, and although not always very sensible by common standards, somehow brilliant.

A cat wandered through the garden. My father remarked, 'I used to have cats. Well, me and some other people. You could say I had a *paw*tial share.'

Once, when I asked him how he was, he answered, 'No wonders, but signs.'

And then there were phrases plucked out of the blue, unreal as words from a dream: 'Life doesn't get any easier without problems.'

The wit and wisdom of August Geiger. The only shame is that language is slowly draining out of him, that breathtaking sentences are becoming rarer and rarer. To think what's lost – that hurts. It's as if I were watching my father bleed to death in slow motion. Life slowly seeps out of him, drop by drop. A person's personality trickles out, drop by drop. It's still intact, the feeling that this is my father, the man who helped bring me up.

But the moments when I no longer recognise the father I once had are becoming more frequent, especially in the evenings.

Evening gives a taste of what mornings will soon bring, for with night comes fear. That is when, restless and helpless, my father wanders around like an old king in his exile. Everything he sees is frightening, everything sways, is unstable, threatens to dissolve in the next instant. And nothing feels like home.

I've been sitting for a while in the kitchen, typing up notes on my laptop. The television is on in the living room and my father, hearing voices coming from there, tiptoes across the floorboards, listens and murmurs to himself a number of times, 'None of my business.'

He then comes into the kitchen and pretends to watch me as I write. But, glancing to the side, I notice he needs help.

'Wouldn't you like to watch some TV?' I ask.

'Why bother?'

'Well, it would be fun.'

'I'd rather go home.'

'You are home.'

'Where are we?'

I give his house number and the street.

'All right, but I was never here much.'

'You built the house in the late fifties and you've lived here ever since.'

He makes a face. He's not satisfied with this information. He scratches his neck.

'I believe you, conditionally. And now I want to go home.'

I look at him. Although he is trying to hide his confusion, you can see how difficult it is for him. He's jumpy. Sweat glistens on his forehead. The sight of this man on the verge of panic shakes me.

His terrifying homeless feeling is a symptom of the illness. I can best explain it to myself like this: because of their inner disintegration, people with dementia no longer feel secure and so they long for a place where they will feel secure again. Yet since their confusion cannot be shaken off anywhere, however familiar the place, even in their own beds they aren't at home.

To echo Marcel Proust: the true paradises are those we have lost. A change of location doesn't help, except as a distraction, and singing serves that purpose just as well, if not better. Singing is more fun. People with dementia love to sing. Singing is emotional – a home outside the tangible world.

It's often said that people with dementia are like small children. Almost all the writing on the subject makes use of the metaphor, which is annoying, because it's impossible for an adult to *regress* to childhood, while it's in a child's nature to *progress*. A child develops new abilities; someone affected by dementia loses theirs. When you spend time with children, you gain a keen eye for every step forward; with dementia, for every loss. The truth is that age gives nothing back. It's a helter-skelter downward slide and one of our greatest worries is that old age can last too long.

I turn the CD player on. My sister Helga bought a collection of classic folk songs for such occasions, such as *Hoch auf dem gelben Wagen* and *Zogen einst fünf wilde Schwäne.* Often the trick works. We warble away for half an hour. He gets so wrapped up in the singing that I have to laugh. My father starts laughing, too, and as it happens to be time for bed, I seize the moment and steer him towards his bedroom. He is now in good spirits, although with no better sense of time, space, or what's going on. At the moment that doesn't bother him.

'Not to win, but to endure is all,' I think, and from this day on I'm at least as exhausted as my father. I tell him what he has to do, until he is wearing his pyjamas. He slips under the covers all by himself and says, 'So long as I have a place to sleep.'

He looks around, lifts a hand, and greets someone whom only he can see. 'It's liveable,' he comments. 'Actually, it's pretty nice.'

How are you, Dad?

Well, actually, I'm fine. But 'fine' in quotation marks, because I'm in no position to judge.

Do you ever think about the passing of time?

Time passing? I don't actually mind whether it passes quickly or slowly. I'm not hard to please with these things.

The shadow of the onset still haunts me, although less intensely as the years go by. When I look out of the window onto the frosty orchard below and think about what happened to us, I'm overcome with the sense of a wrong step taken long ago.

Our father's illness started in such a confusingly slow way that it was difficult to assign changes their true meanings. Things crept up on us, like Death in an old legend, hiding in the hallway and rattling his bones. We heard the noise and thought it was the wind in our ever-more-dilapidated house.

The earliest signs of the illness were there in the mid-nineties, but we didn't manage to interpret them. Thinking back on the renovation work on the terrace flat, I can only shake my head bitterly: my father smashed to pieces the concrete covers of the disused septic tank, because he couldn't lift them up and replace them over the opening. That was not the first time I believed he was making my life difficult on purpose. We shouted at each other. As the work continued, I often left the house fearing that when I returned, I'd be in for more nasty shocks.

Then there was the time a Swiss radio producer visited. That too is a day that has stuck in my memory. It was autumn 1997, shortly after my first novel had come out. He came to record a chapter that I would read aloud, so I asked my father not to make any noise that afternoon. Scarcely had the session begun before we heard a hammering from my father's workshop, which lasted as long as the producer's mic was on. Throughout my reading, I felt a deep anger towards my father – hatred, in fact, because of his lack of consideration. I avoided him for days, didn't speak a word to him. The word on the tip of my tongue was 'sabotage'.

And when did Peter, my older brother, get married? That was 1993. Our father got an upset stomach at the wedding reception, because he lost all sense of moderation and after the meal's many courses devoured a dozen pieces of cake. Late that night he dragged himself home and had to spend a painful few days in bed. He was afraid of dying, but no one felt sorry for him because, as we thought, it was his own fault. No one noticed that he was gradually losing everyday skills.

The illness caught him in its net, gradually, subtly. Our father was already deeply entangled in it, without our noticing.

While we children were misinterpreting the signs, it must have been absolute torment for him to see himself change – and to fear that he was being taken over by something hostile, against which he couldn't defend himself. He never commented on it. He wasn't open enough to do that, nor able to share his emotions. It wasn't in his character. It never had been and it was too late to change now. What made matters worse was that he had passed on to his children this lack of openness, which is why there was no real attempt from our side either. No one made the effort. We let things run their course. 'Well, yes, he's acting odd at times, but didn't he always?' This behaviour was actually normal for him.

*

At first, any peculiarities on his part really did look like the understandable effects of the new circumstances in which he found himself. He was ageing and his wife had left him after thirty years of marriage. It was easy to assume that this was the root of his apathy.

The separation had been tough on him. He had been dead set against divorce, partly because he wanted to stay with my mother, and partly because he believed some things were absolutely binding. He had not fully realised that certain conventions had become unable to bear the heavy loads they carried. In stark contrast to today's flexibility about such things, my father held to a decision he had made decades ago and didn't want to break his vows. In this respect he belonged to a different generation from his wife, who was fifteen years younger. For her, it was not her reputation or word that was at stake, but her life and the possibility of finding happiness elsewhere. My mother left their house, while my father clung inwardly to the dead relationship, faithful to what he had already lost.

As if something inside him had snapped, my mother's departure led to a period of brooding and inaction. He even stopped looking after the garden, although he knew that his children were very busy with their jobs and struggled under the extra burden. He freed himself from practically all obligations. There was no trace of the enthusiasm with which he used to dive into projects. He announced that it was the young ones' turn now – he'd already worked enough in his life.

We were annoyed by his excuses, and excuses they were, although for something other than what we suspected. We thought his failings were a result of doing nothing. But it was the other way around: the doing nothing was a result of his failings. As even small tasks were now too much for him, and as he knew he was losing control, he surrendered all responsibility.

Instead of watering the tomato plants every day, he spent his time playing patience and watching television. I remember how his monotonous pleasures left a terrible taste in my mouth. At a time when I was getting my career going, it seemed to me that dull indifference ruled his life. 'Playing patience and watching television? That's hardly enough for a life,' I thought, and made no bones about my opinion. I pleaded with him, I teased and provoked him, I talked about inertia and the need for action. But even the most stubborn attempts to tear him out of his numbness failed dismally. With the look of a horse standing motionless in a storm, he would let my attacks wash over him. Then he'd go back to his routine.

If, back then, I hadn't needed to work several months each year as a sound man at the Bregenz Festival, earning the money that writing didn't bring my way, I would have avoided the family home. I only had to be back for a few days before a deep misery descended on me. It was the same for my siblings. Gradually everyone left home. We children scattered. Life got tougher for our father.

That was how we felt in the year 2000. Not only was the illness eating away at our father's brain, it was also eating at the image that I had formed of him. Throughout my childhood and youth I had been proud to be his son. Now I was increasingly thinking of him as a halfwit.

Jacques Derrida was not wrong when he said that when you write, you are always asking for forgiveness.

*

Aunt Hedwig tells a story of a visit she and Emil – the eldest of my father's six brothers – once paid him. Emil had brought hair clippers and a towel, although Aunt Hedwig no longer remembers whether my father let Emil cut his hair. It was mid-afternoon. To Aunt Hedwig's surprise, there was a plate with leftover tomato sauce on the coffee table by the sofa. Later my father dropped a glass, and when he looked helplessly at it, Aunt Hedwig offered to clean up the shards. She asked him where he kept the dustpan and brush. He couldn't recall. Looking at her, his eyes suddenly filled with tears. That was the moment when she knew.

They didn't talk about it. Silently my father fought with himself. He didn't attempt to explain anything. He didn't attempt to escape – not until the pilgrimage to Lourdes.

That was in 1998, with Maria, the eldest of his three sisters, Erich, his youngest surviving brother, and Waltraud, his sister-in-law. My father, who hadn't gone on a single holiday with his wife and children because – so he always said – he had seen the world during the war, now set off on a comparatively long journey with the faint hope of healing.

And then to stand there with an empty smile and pray at night and – as if the night prayers had no power – to do it again in the morning.

Maria, who by then was none too steady on her feet, apparently said to him, 'You walk for me, and I'll think for you.'

*

What we don't understand terrifies us most. Which is why the situation improved for us once the signs accumulated that our father was affected by more than just forgetfulness and a lack of motivation. When everyday tasks presented him with insoluble problems, absent-mindedness could no longer be invoked as an excuse. It was impossible to keep fooling ourselves. Dressing himself in the morning, our father would only put on half his clothes, or put them on backwards or put on four sets. At lunch he would stick a frozen pizza, still in its plastic wrap, into the oven, and put his socks in the fridge. There came a time when we knew our father was affected by dementia and not just letting himself go – though we were slow to grasp the full extent of the horror.

For years the thought hadn't even crossed my mind. My childhood image of my father blocked it out. As absurd as it sounds, dementia was the last thing I expected from him.

*

Our insight into the true situation came as a relief to all. Now there was an acceptable explanation for the chaos of the last few years. We no longer felt so utterly devastated, though our relief was tinged by the bitterness of knowing we had wasted so much time fighting a phantom – time that we should have been using much more wisely. If we had been cleverer, more attentive and more engaged, we would have spared our father and ourselves a lot of trouble. We would have taken better care of him and found time to ask more questions before it was too late.

*

The onset of the illness was a terrible time, a complete failure. What's more, it was the time of the greatest losses.

By that I mean the losses of both my father's memories and the physical disappearance of items that had been important to him. His bicycle from the fifties, a three-speed with curving handlebars and a leather saddle with squeaky springs. For decades, even on snow and ice, my father had ridden it to the parish offices where he had started as a clerk at the age of twenty-six. Lost. The headshot that had been taken right after the war, of a young man who weighed not much over six stone. Lost. My father had carried the photo around for almost sixty years in his wallet, along with a photo of his mother. Things he treasured.

I told a friend that seeing my barely nineteen-year-old father in this photo, just a few days after his discharge from a Russian military hospital, had made a strong impression on me. At that hospital, he recovered from dysentery, more by luck than medical care, after weeks in unimaginable conditions and on the verge of the grave.

He used to enjoy showing people the photo. In it he had very short hair, bony features, and a look that was hard to fathom but suggested both clarity and fear in his darkly gleaming eyes, which were sympathetic. You wouldn't tease a man for keeping a photo like that in his wallet instead of one of the wife and kids.

Before I left for Wolfurt, the same friend urged me to make a copy of the photo. She was surprised I hadn't done so yet. That was in 2004. Coming from Berlin, I arrived at my father's house in the afternoon. While my father was sitting in Peter and Ursula's garden, watching his grandchildren play, as he did just about every afternoon, I patted down all his jackets and trousers, rummaged through drawers and wardrobes, just as I had done decades ago as a child, when I snooped around the house. This time my snooping was in vain. I called Helga to ask if she knew where our father's wallet was. She said that it hadn't been around for years, because he'd lost it. I still remember how devastated I was, how angry – angry at myself, angry at all of us – because we hadn't done something in time.

I mentioned the photo to my father that evening. He came up with a far-fetched story about being in Egypt and in Greece, where his trousers had been stolen, and along with them his wallet.

'How? What? Where?' I asked, severely shaken. Suddenly it was clear that not just a photo had been discarded, but also my father's knowledge of his past.

'Dad, you say you were in Egypt?'

'Not voluntarily, of course. But as part of the evacuation of children during the war.'

'And how did you find it?' I asked reluctantly.

'It was boring.' He shrugged. 'I didn't see or experience anything. I was there as a nobody, a no-good no-hoper.'

How was your childhood, Dad?

Good. Harmless. What we had was all a bit primitive, in terms of its nature, quantity, as well as its effectiveness.

Do you often think about it?

I can remember some things, but I no longer know everything. I think I've left all that behind.

What do you recall about your father?

Nothing right now.

But you had a father?

Yes, of course.

So he wasn't anyone particularly important in your life?

ie didn't have many important thoughts.
nough.

ier?

My __ er! From her I learnt to be humble. She was an unassuming person, always friendly and ready to help. She liked everyone._

Children called August are rare these days. And yet the name served my father well for eight and a half decades. Only his classmates shortened it to 'Gustl'. Everyone else – parents, siblings, work colleagues, wife – used his full name throughout his life. August.

The third of ten children, he was born on 4 July 1926. His parents owned a small farm in Wolfurt, a Rhine Valley village in Austria's westernmost region, the Vorarlberg. Due to the local laws of inheritance, the district has no large farms. My father's parents had three cows, an orchard, a ploughed field, a meadow, a small wood, a licence to distil three hundred litres of schnapps, and a beehive. A family with so many children couldn't live off that. Adolf Geiger, their *Dätt* ('dad' in the local Alemannic dialect), brought in a salary working for the nascent electric power industry. He rode his bike through the villages of the Lower Rhine Valley and read people's meters.

When Dätt got a flat from a stray horseshoe nail, he would leave his bike in front of the house for one of his kids, normally August, to patch the tyre. I also used to put my bike in front of the house for my father to patch. And just as my father had to obey his parents, it was later expected that he would obey his children. His children were born into a different world and thought they knew best how things should be done.

Dätt was good with numbers, but otherwise not particularly gifted nor physically strong. He preferred giving orders to working, because everyone else in the family was more skilled and soon also stronger than he was, and he didn't want to embarrass himself in front of his wife and children. For the same reason, Dätt never explained how to do or make anything. He just ordered that it be done. That way he avoided ever being told how to do it better.

Dätt was an authoritarian. He often lost control and slapped his children. Nevertheless, his children's strategy wasn't always one of avoidance. When they could no longer bear the nonsense that he spouted, they would argue with him (so say Maria and Paul).

The older children saw Dätt as a nuisance and steered clear of him when possible. They set off for Mass three minutes before or after him, but never with him. From the edge of the family he made an effort to have a better relationship with the younger children. He behaved better with them, played board games like Fox and Geese, and took them on long walks. He was already older by then. But the boxings he gave their ears still echo in their stories.

Once, Dätt had his son Emil, then fourteen, carry him on his back over the Schwarzach stream. That was in 1937. He couldn't be bothered to take his shoes off, apparently.

And they say he read a lot. But along with his slapping, reading was not something that he passed on to his children. Their mother's personality traits were more infectious.

Their *Mam*, as they called her, was cleverer than Dätt. That's what my father said when the threads of memory still tied him to such things. Warm-hearted and friendly, she was a slim but strong woman with well-defined biceps. Her father was the blacksmith in Wolfurt. In her youth, before she started to work as an embroiderer, she helped out in the smithy, because she had no brothers and because her father noticed that she was a quick learner.

The smithy is up on a hill at the edge of the woods, behind the schloss, and it has a large waterwheel. Before and after World War I, a truck from Dornbirn would leave the materials the smith had ordered at the end of the road leading to the castle, and after school the smith's five daughters would carry the long iron bars up the steep road.

Mam was a quiet woman who hated it when people fussed over her. She saw life as the preparation for heaven. Her children speak of her with nothing but respect, which is probably why they have so few stories to tell about her. It was said that Theresia Geiger was one of the three hardest-working women in the village, so much so that she often felt like a servant girl, and wouldn't have been worse off if she'd continued working for her father at the anvil, hammering iron until it glowed. There was farm work to attend to, and there were always little children whose nappies needed changing. Every evening she would be soaked from wringing water out of washed cloth nappies. Sometimes she would lie down on the sofa during the day and ask one of her children to wake her up in five minutes. They just let their mother sleep.

When they went to gather fruit, Mam would say before they set out, 'God bless our work.'

Irene, my father's youngest sister, still remembers that when she goes out to the fields.

For almost two decades, a large fruit crate with a small child inside stood in the field as they worked. The children learnt to walk in that fruit crate. Dätt's initials were burned into the wood: A.G. The brand was courtesy of his father-in-law, the smith, whose speciality was creating branding irons – letters and symbols. He had sold them widely, from Hungary to Paris, and yet he remained poor, up on the castle mound from where you could see over into Appenzell in Switzerland, across Lake Constance to Lindau and, if the weather was good, as far as Friedrichshafen.

Theresia Geiger would say to her children, 'Don't come home too late, and if you do, then do it quietly please, so I don't wake up.'

The daily routine barely changed at all. Mam woke all the children early in the morning, rousing them several times until they were finally up. Often the children had to run to school, because they had cut it too close with their timing. They didn't have great footwear. In the winter, snow stuck to their wooden soles, so that they had to stop and keep knocking off the clumps. The wooden shoes crunched through the snow, which often fell around St Nicholas Day and lay on the ground until spring.

At breakfast they dunked *Riebel*, the traditional pan-fried cornmeal porridge eaten by the poor, in a bowl of warm milk. Mam and Dätt drank coffee. Only Datt got honey, except on Sundays, when there was honey for all. After the meal, prayers were said for unfortunate souls.

In that family, the children weren't brought up, but 'kept' – the same as for cows. It was the children's task to keep the cows, and the parents' task to keep the children.

By today's standards the children didn't have a balanced diet. They had almost no vegetables and very little meat, but a lot of milk, bread and lard. They longed for the first fruit of the year. Sometimes in summer, one child would wake at five in the morning and creep outside to see if any early 'hay' pears had fallen. The children each ferreted away little troves of their finds, so that they wouldn't have to share with their brothers and sisters.

The privations of their childhood were not extreme, given the general conditions then. It was harder to bear the scarcity of affection and attention from their parents. Because of the large number of children, demand far exceeded supply. Everything had to be shared many ways.

As soon as a child could hold a tool, their help was expected. The little ones looked after the littlest while the older children worked. The horse that had been borrowed from the neighbour had to be rid of its flies so it wouldn't bolt. The children were sent out to the boggy patch to gather acorns for the pigs in the sty. Josef, the fourth of the seven sons, was once found unconscious under an oak, because he had fallen out of the tree. When the grass was mowed, the children would pick out the plants that the cows shouldn't eat: hogweed and curly dock. They used a handcart to take the apples to market in Bregenz and Mam would follow later on her bike. On the way home my father and Paul, who was a year younger, couldn't resist playing around. They would take turns sitting in the handcart while the other one was the horse. Their nailed clogs clacked on the cobbles. Back then children still owned the roads.

They understood the phrase *putting your back into it* quite literally. The boys would pull the hay wagon and garner taunts from the girls: 'Spare the horses, use an ass!'

There was boys' work and girls' work. The boys had to clean out the barn and the girls got up at five in the morning to weed the field before school.

Once a storm completely flattened the field. The children spent a day with wire and stakes, tying the maize plants up. The family relied on the corn for their daily Riebel.

The family was largely self-sufficient, buying only bread, flour, sugar and salt – the absolute necessities. Toilet paper was cut in strips of a hand's breadth from old newspapers. This too was a chore for the children. One of them would sit at the parlour table and tear up the paper.

Paper was needed to light the stove too. There was almost no waste. The family had a stove, a dungheap and a pig.

My father would have liked to have stayed frugal his whole life. It was a deeply rooted part of his farm upbringing, and it stuck, much to the dissatisfaction of his wife and children, who had grown up in a world of disposable consumer goods. His ability to make do and mend, as well as his willingness – picked up from his parents – to delay the satisfaction of his needs, or to deny himself completely those needs: these traits belong to a culture that is disappearing.

The large house had a still in the cellar. As a child, I would sit on an upturned bucket or a block of wood and watch the schnapps being made. I loved the crackling of the stove fire and the drip-drop trickle of alcohol as it fell into the large-bellied bottles – the aromatic scent of schnapps mixing with the smell of men working hard. And outside, the cooling marc in the ditch, the mist in the bare wintery branches of the pear tree.

For my father and his siblings, distilling had the benefit of providing hot water. The water was fed through to
a big wooden tub in the neighbouring workshop that
also contained the chicken coop behind wire mesh.
About ten times a year it was like a spaghetti western
scene – the scent of spirits, the clucking of hens, the
farmer's naked offspring in the water. The rest of the
time everyone washed in the kitchen, in the house's
only sink, using cold water.

My father held stubbornly to the way of life he had
grown up with. Even as an adult, he would wash at the
sink. Bending deep over it, puffing and blowing, he would
slap water onto his face, spraying it for yards around.
He would bore deep into his ears with a washcloth on
his index finger, waggling it so violently that it hurt
just to watch.

That is the meagre harvest gleaned from occasional
comments – a few stalks left on a mowed field.

*

In 1938 came the Anschluss. The family had always been
among the village's public supporters of the Christian
Social Party. Dätt and Mam saw their Catholicism as
more than just something for Sundays. Additionally,
the family didn't own any business interests that could
have benefited from the new political situation. Thanks
to the small farm and Dätt's job, the family was largely
sheltered from crises. 'Guns are loaded by the Devil,'

Mam said. And when his brother-in-law became the Nazi mayor, Dätt – who always did just as he damn well pleased – went back to using the distanced *Sie* word for 'you' when addressing him, instead of *Du*.

The family didn't talk politics. Everyone's mouth was full at mealtimes, and there was no time for sitting around afterwards – chop-chop! They had to eat up and get back to work. Then the order came for Emil, the eldest son, to join the Hitler Youth. He refused, saying he couldn't, as he was with the Red Cross. When Emil was threatened with expulsion from the business academy if he didn't change his mind, Dätt didn't shirk confrontation. Emil was allowed to stay in school, but the family's child benefit was cut off for all eight children. The family had no further trouble, however, unlike the next-door neighbours, who were shamed by a sign on their house that read '*Diese familie ist gegen das deutsche Volk*,' or, 'This family is against the German people.'

Paul remembers the lower-case *f* in *familie*, when in correct German it should be a capital *F*. He was eleven or twelve and had stood in front of the sign for a good while, surprised at the mistake. A newly married man and woman lived in that house. When the woman died at the age of ninety-four, my father took over her nursing home room. That's how people's lives are linked in a small village.

When the war started, my father and all his school-age siblings were either at the business academy or the grammar school. They were given more than a basic education because on the one hand, their parents respected education as an alternative to their small-scale farming (which would have, at most, been able to provide a living for one child), and on the other hand they took joy in their offspring's talents. They also liked the fact that schoolchildren could help at home more than apprentices could. Nobody in the family objected to schooling except Robert, the third-youngest son, who dropped out because he was afraid that they wanted to make a priest of him.

*

Because it was wartime, my father had to take early graduation exams in February 1944 and was conscripted: a mere seventeen-year-old grammar-school boy from a farming family, an unworldly altar boy with little life experience – neither a child nor an adult, neither military nor civilian, as Bulgakov called such schoolboy soldiers.

He was transferred from the Labour Service to the Wehrmacht in the summer of 1944. It was a similar story for his brother Emil, three years older, and Paul, one year younger. Back home the family was now forced to follow political developments more closely, concerned about their conscripted brothers and sons, the boys. When they hadn't heard anything for weeks, 'What's happened?'

Emil was lucky. He quickly fell into American hands in Africa and spent the rest of the war as an interpreter in Montana. Letters from him arrived home after a while, so the family knew he was safe.

Paul was captured in 1945 in Italy by troops from New Zealand. In the POW camp near Bari, he found ways to earn a little extra money on the side. He made needles from fencing wire and would knit caps from unravelled pullover sleeves, selling them to fellow prisoners who either suffered in the sun or simply wanted to look good. He wore his own cap for a long time after the war.

As Paul was only seventeen, he was sent home in the summer of 1945. He didn't tell people he was coming. Arriving completely unnoticed, he went to see the three cows in the barn first, and then to the still, where cousin Rudolf was making schnapps. Rudolf climbed up the steps to the kitchen ahead of him, where Mam was working. Not many days earlier she had lost her tenth child, a boy, just hours after the birth. The umbilical cord had got caught around the baby's neck.

'Got a soldier here looking for somewhere to stay, Theres,' Rudolf told her.

She had hesitated, because the house was full, even with three sons gone. Then Paul stepped forward out of the shadows and tears started to run down his cheeks.

At first things seemed to work out for my father too. During his training he was twice sent home on sick leave because of a stubborn infection in his lower right arm. Soon after, he offered to go home and fetch 'the club' some schnapps for the Christmas festivities. He spent two Advent weeks in Wolfurt. But then, in

February 1945, he was sent to the Eastern Front to be an eighteen-year-old trucker without a driver's licence. In Upper Silesia he got into a serious accident when a horse-drawn cart didn't get out of his way on a highway. His horn broken and brakes useless because of the ice on the road, he steered the truck down the embankment. The truck rolled over several times. When his superior threatened to send my father in front of a war tribunal for sabotage, my father noted the fact that he had no driver's licence and shouldn't have been driving at all.

When the general disintegration of the army was apparent, he took himself off and tried with a few other Austrians to reach the American forces. Perhaps out of homesickness, the group went in the wrong direction – instead of going west, they went south, right through Bohemia, taking the shortest route towards home, but also towards the Russians. They were already on Austrian soil, in the Kamp Valley, when their hopes of a quick return were dashed.

When my father would later claim that he saw the world during the war, he didn't mean the war so much as the time after it. His punishment as a POW was to move the spoils of war for his captors. Once, during a meal, he found a bone in the soup that was obviously rotten, but in his hunger he gnawed away at it. The next day he had dysentery and very soon he weighed no more than six stone. He spent the next four weeks in an army hospital at the edge of Bratislava, in conditions that I knew nothing of until a few months ago. He never once mentioned those four weeks. My father's tales would start with the day when the Soviets let him go, 'because I wasn't worth anything to them any more.'

Together with some other Austrians, he was taken by a Red Army soldier to the Austrian-Slovakian border on the Morava river near Hainburg.

'Goodbye, Austrians!' were the Red Army soldier's parting words. Even now, sometimes my father murmurs these words when he is deep in thought.

The trip back to Vorarlberg took another three weeks, with obstacles at every turn. My father had neither the money nor the papers he needed to go from the Soviet to the American zone. He didn't want to have a photo taken for an identity card, because it would have taken two weeks for the film to be developed. Plagued by homesickness, he hoped for the opportunity to cross the border illegally.

He refused the beds that were offered to him, because he knew he had lice. He slept in the skittle alley of an inn and on farmers' hay.

After six days of waiting in Urfahr, some fellow Vorarl-bergers smuggled him across the Danube to Linz under the seat of a Red Cross vehicle. He was deloused by the Americans.

Now he had his photo taken, because there was a photographer in Linz who could develop the film quickly. This was the very photo that he carried around for almost sixty years in his wallet.

On the train, somewhere past Innsbruck, he met some people from Wolfurt and asked them for bread. In Lauterach, where he got out, he met a cousin, who didn't recognise him at first because of his short hair and all the weight he had lost. The cousin accompanied him home.

I can only imagine my father's feelings when he returned after his long absence. Even when I come from Vienna, there's a joy that wells up when I read the names of the stations after the Arlberg Tunnel, as if they were part of a poem: Langen, Wald, Dalaas, Braz, Bings, Bludenz.

My father came home in the second week of September, on the ninth, when the light was once again golden and the third hay harvest was about to be brought in, ahead of the pear and apple harvest. And in October, as if nothing had happened, he was at a desk again at the business academy.

Or was there more to it than that?

What no one knew at the time was that this nineteen-year-old would never again open himself up to the world. That was over for good. He must have sworn to himself in the hospital never to leave home again, if he were ever to make it back from his long, slow journey. His earlier ambition of studying electrical engineering was gone. Facts change feelings.

I still remember how difficult a topic holidays were when I was growing up. My father would say a hundred times over that Wolfurt was lovely enough for him. At the time such phrases seemed like patent disguises for his inertia. And they may very well have been excuses, but if so, then just in part. It was only much later that I came to understand that behind my father's refusal lay a trauma, and that in our hearts, things never end; for this reason, my father's behaviour was what it was. He took these precautions to ensure that he would never be in danger again. He didn't want to be so far from home a second time.

It's a strange irony that he did, of course, end up in a situation many years later in which he wanted almost daily to get home – because he had forgotten he was already there.

Look, Dad, this is the garden wall you made with your own hands.

True. I'll take it home with me.

You can't take it with you.

Nothing easier.

It can't be done, Dad.

Let me show you.

Oh, come on, Dad – seriously?! You can't do it. And here's another question for you – tell me how you plan to go home, when you're already home.

I don't quite follow.

You're home but you want to go home. You can't go home when you're already home.

That's true, objectively speaking.

So?

I'm not nearly as interested in all that as you are.

Our early failures behind us, we had become more understanding with our father, although each new day still kept us on our toes with its own surprises. We didn't look back much, always forwards, for the illness kept giving us new challenges. We were beginners, trying to maintain a semblance of control over our lives, but without basic knowledge or skills.

Our father took to wandering. Mainly he walked to my older brother Peter's house. Peter lives across the street and has three daughters. But increasingly his excursions took him beyond that familiar radius – sometimes in the middle of the night, barely clothed, with a frightened look in his eye. Once we couldn't find him because he had strayed into one of the children's bedrooms in his house and laid down in a bed. Sometimes he rummaged through wardrobes and was then surprised when my brother Werner's trousers didn't fit him. There came a day when we wrote *August* on his door and locked the neighbouring rooms.

Often he had blood on his head or cuts on his knees when he came back from a wander to his childhood home. He would stumble on the steep and overgrown hill. Once he forced his way into his parents' old home and suddenly appeared at the top of the stairs in front of his sister-in-law, asking after his brother Erich. When I was a child, the latch on the front door could easily be opened by sticking a finger through a hole in the wood. My father must have tried to do so again and again, not knowing that the latch didn't work any more. The futility of his efforts threw him so much that he decided to break down the door.

My sister recalls how he would answer the phone, but a minute later would have forgotten the message he was supposed to pass on. And of course, if one of his possessions was missing, it was always *the others* who had taken or stolen it. When we asked him where something was, he knew nothing and reacted indignantly to the suggestion that he might have had anything to do with its disappearance. His electric shaver, for which we had been desperately searching, turned up in the microwave. He had been losing his front door key so regularly that my mother not only tied the key to his trousers, she sewed it on. That didn't seem right to him, however, so he would tug and pull at it.

He developed obsessions. His most stubborn bugbear was with the birch that stood near the house and which Hurricane Lothar had knocked to a sharp angle. Dozens of times a day, our father, either pointing at the tree that continued to grow to ever-greater heights or looking at the approaching clouds, would ask whether the birch would withstand the next storm or fall on the house. The electric meter was never far from his thoughts either. He would check it manically. I can still hear the regular click of the magnetic catch as he opened and shut the cupboard with the meter. When the house was rattling with cold on winter mornings, we knew that our father had been messing with one of the switches again. Who was to blame? *The others*, of course.

Dätt, we had heard, had also been a keen energy saver. When he joined his family for breakfast and thought it was already bright enough outside, he would turn off the light, saying, 'You'll find your mouths easily enough.'

Little stories like that.

Dätt had always been careful to ensure that the curtains didn't hang in front of the windows. He used to push them all the way to the side, to let in the most light possible. He had been very frugal – perhaps the only characteristic that had been wholly passed on to his children.

Now our father would constantly think about energy consumption, too. His brain at this time was like a barrel organ, always playing the same tune.

But then one day, the obsessions disappeared. It was a little spooky. Our father started being creative.

For a long time we had been dealing with his forgetfulness and lost abilities, but now the illness started to uncover new skills. Our father, who had always been an honest man, developed a real talent for excuses. He could find an excuse quicker than a mouse its hole. His manner of speaking changed and suddenly displayed a spontaneous elegance that I'd never noticed before. And what he said had such a striking internal logic that we didn't know whether to be astonished, to laugh, or to cry.

'What beautiful weather!' I remarked once, as we stood by his house with a view of the Gebhardsberg summit, across the Bregenzer Ache river, and to the Känzele's slopes.

My father looked around, thought about what I had said, and replied, 'I could predict the weather reliably from home, but from here I can't. As I'm no longer at home, it's become impossible.'

'The climate here is almost the same as down there,' I said in surprise, as our house is only fifty yards up the hill from his parents'.

'Yes, that's just it. You see what a difference that can make!' He thought for a moment, adding, 'And what's more, things don't turn out well when you all meddle in my weather.'

His new talents were most evident when he would get stressed trying to find his way home. It must have been around 2004 when he suddenly stopped recognising his own house. It happened surprisingly, shockingly, quickly. We could hardly take it in. For a long time we refused to accept that our father had forgotten something as fundamental as this.

One day my sister couldn't listen to his insistent pleading any longer. Every five minutes he said that he was expected at home. It was unbearable, or at least that's how it felt to us at the time. Helga went out into the street with him and announced, 'This is your house!'

'No, it's not my house,' he replied.

'Then tell me where you live.'

He gave the right house number and street name.

Helga pointed triumphantly to the sign by the front door on which was written the house number, and asked, 'And what does this say?'

He read out the number he had mentioned before.

'So what can we conclude?' Helga asked.

'That someone stole the sign and screwed it on here,' replied our father without blinking an eye. It was a fantastical idea, but one that made sense in its way.

'Why would someone steal our house sign and screw it onto their house?' asked Helga crossly.

'Good question. That's just what people are like.'

There was a tone of regret in his statement, but he was completely untroubled by his improbable explanation.

Another time, when I asked him if he recognised his own furniture, he replied, 'Yes, now I do!'

'I should hope so,' I said, somewhat condescendingly.

He looked at me disappointedly and explained, 'You know, it's not as easy as you think. Other people have furniture like this. You never know.'

His answer was so perfectly logical and, in its way, convincing, that it really got my back up. It wasn't possible.

Why were we having this discussion at all, when he was capable of such ideas? Surely I could expect that someone intelligent enough to tease out such nuances could recognise his own house. But, sadly, he couldn't.

Not that he was always open to persuasion. He might instead examine all the room's details suspiciously, ultimately arriving at the conclusion that it had been rearranged to trick him. Such episodes reminded me of the thriller *36 Hours* with James Garner and Eva Marie Saint, in which Garner plays an American secret service agent with important information about the Allies' invasion. The Nazis lure him into a trap and drug him. When he wakes up the next day, he is told that he's in an American military hospital and that the war was won years ago. They tell him that he suffered amnesia. The deception is perfect except for one minor injury that the officer had received and which – although, supposedly, years have passed – still has not healed.

For years such inconsistencies must have been my father's daily experience. He was living in constant distrust of his family's ostensibly plausible explanations. As he said, 'Home looks a lot like this – just a little different.'

*

He often sat alone in the living room, sighing. Each time he did, it frightened me to see how fragile he seemed, how abandoned. He had changed. His worried expression no longer conveyed despair at how much he forgot, but instead the utter homelessness of a person for whom the whole world has become foreign. That feeling of abandonment, combined with his conviction that simply changing locations would cure it, often stalemated him for days.

When he said he was going home, it was not really in opposition to the place he wanted to leave, but rather to the situation in which he felt uncomfortable. And yet he took the illness with him wherever he went – even to his parents' house. His childhood home was within spitting distance of his own, but it remained an unattainable destination – not because he couldn't walk there, but because his arrival never had the effect he ultimately desired. No matter where he went, the impossibility of feeling at home stuck to the soles of his feet. Ill as he was, he couldn't see how his condition affected his perception of location. But every day, his family could see what true homesickness was.

We felt so sorry for him. More than anything, we would have loved him to recover his sense of being at home. In a way, that would have signalled that he was in remission, but that's only possible with cancer and not Alzheimer's.

The situation became somewhat easier two years later, as if to confirm the platitude that things get worse before they get better.

And only years later did I realise that the desire to go home is a deep part of being human. Intuitively, as a cure for a frightening and inescapable illness, our father had named a place where he would feel safe once he reached it. He called this comforting place 'home'; believers call it 'heaven'.

What Ovid wrote in exile – that home is where people understand your language – was true for our father in no less existential a way. Because he increasingly struggled to follow conversations or to recognise faces, he felt as though he was in exile. The people speaking to him, even his own siblings and children, were strangers, because the things they said were confusing and strange. His gradual conclusion that his home wasn't *here* made perfect sense. And it was also completely logical that he would keep wanting to go home, convinced that only then would life return to normal.

*

'I washed my hands here,' my father once said. 'Was I allowed to?'

'Yes, it's your house and your sink.'

He looked at me in astonishment and, smiling embarrassedly, said, 'Good Lord, hopefully I won't forget that again!'

That's dementia. Or perhaps I should say that's life – the stuff of life.

*

Alzheimer's, like everything of significance, shines a light on much beyond itself. Human characteristics and society's mores are enlarged by the illness as if under a magnifying glass. The world is confusing to all of us, and when you look at it with a clear eye, you see that the biggest difference between the healthy and the sick is simply the degree to which they are able to conceal the confusion. Underneath, chaos roils.

Even for us generally healthy people, the order in our heads is a fiction of our reason. Alzheimer's opens our eyes to the complex skills we use just to get through each day. In addition, Alzheimer's takes on symbolic value in our society, in which it's no longer possible to see the overall picture or to synthesise all the available knowledge. Ceaseless change can be disorientating and lead to fears about the future. To talk about Alzheimer's is to talk about the illness of our century. By chance, my father's life also reflects this development. It began in an era built on strong pillars – family, religion, power structures, ideologies, gender roles, the fatherland – and at the end of it came his illness, at a time when those structures had been toppled.

As this realisation dawned on me, I started to feel ever closer to my father.

*

But at the time I didn't get it. I'm not always the quickest of people. I blundered on, because I didn't want to stop believing that I could keep my father connected to reality.

When he said that his mother was waiting for him, I asked the harmless sounding question, 'How old is your mother?'

'Um, about eighty.'

'And how old are you?'

'Well, I was born in 1926, so I'm – '

'Also about eighty.'

'Right, I know that.'

'Your mother's dead,' I said, sadly.

He pursed his lips, nodded a number of times, and then replied with a contemplative look, 'I *almost* feared as much.'

I carried on fighting for common sense a good while longer. But after I'd had to admit many times how pointless my efforts were, I gave up the battle and once again saw that if you give up, you can win. Was she dead or alive? Who cares? It made no difference. Once I had accepted that my father was reviving the dead a little, and, in so doing, bringing himself a little closer to death, I managed to enter deeper into his suffering.

Now we were all setting off towards a different life and, as much as this different life left my siblings and me uneasy, we all felt a growing sympathy for our father's fate. For years I hadn't been interested in what he did, whether it was playing patience or watching TV, but now I had a renewed interest, not least because I sensed that I might discover something about myself. The question was what.

Daily interactions with my father were exhausting, but they were increasingly leaving me inspired too. The psychological strain continued to be immense, but I noticed that my feelings towards him were changing. His personality seemed to have been rebuilt. It was as if he were like before, just a little changed. And I was changing too. The illness affected all of us.

What's your favourite place, Dad?

Hard to say. I like being out in the street.

What do you do out in the street?

Walk. Run sometimes. But I'm not well saddled. My shoes don't have the right translation.

So, you like being out in the street, although you can't go very fast?

Yes. You see, here inside . . .

Don't you like it here inside?

What am I supposed to do here? I know, the street isn't always right, but it's what I like best, when it's dry. Out there I can look around a bit. That doesn't do anyone any harm.

The illness's onward march was slow but inexorable. Our father could no longer do everyday tasks without danger to himself. He would have been lost without other people's help.

His wife and children no longer lived in the house in the upper field, so he was sent meals on wheels. Soon, his loss of further skills necessitated hourly visits from a mobile care service. In practice, that meant someone came to get him up in the morning, and in the evening someone put him to bed. It was a blessing that he would sleep for so long, although it wasn't clear whether he actually slept deeply for twelve hours or just stayed in bed because he liked the warmth – he, the former farm boy, whose childhood bedroom had been so cold that condensation ran down the walls. When the women from the care service or Ursula, Peter's wife, went into his room just before nine in the morning, he was normally still wrapped up tight in his blanket, although his light had been switched off around nine the previous evening.

Our father would stand around all day in Peter and Ursula's garden, waiting for someone – preferably, his granddaughters – to keep him company. Things couldn't go on like that. He had no sense of the frequency and length of his visits. So we started to look for some hourly help in the afternoons. Liliane, a neighbour whom we trusted, played simple board games with him and took him with her on walks and trips. Ursula would take him to spend one or two days a week at the old people's home as a day visitor. It was a good time and a satisfactory arrangement for everyone.

Helga took over at weekends and Werner kept an eye on my father's house and the gardening. My mother and I would sometimes come from Vienna for a few days or weeks. We slept in the house and took care of everything to give the others a breather. We all found our own ways to cope with the new situation, each of us according to our own strengths and skills. God knows we had other things to do and wished our lives were a little easier. In spite of sharing the workload, right from the start it was a strength-sapping effort.

Even so, the feeling that we were in this together as a family grew. All of us siblings were in the same boat, even if we were taking up different positions.

That was also the time when I suddenly, very suddenly, became a successful author. It was as if success just came rattling down the chimney. Until then I had been praised, but not read. Now attention and invitations flooded in from around the world, and with them came certain advantages, but also the disadvantage that I had to find time for a kind of work I hadn't had before. I hadn't imagined that success would be such a drain on my time, nor did I think it was a good moment to play truant. 'You have to make hay while the sun shines,' my father might have said if these things got through to him by then. Success? Failure? It was all the same to him.

When I graduated and told my father that I wanted to be a writer, he looked at me, grinned, and said, 'I used to scratch things out myself.'

'You did?'

'Yes, out of my nose with one finger.'

I can clearly remember that moment, standing in my father's workshop in front of the shelf of paints and varnishes. He had a knack for saying things in such a way that I could never be angry with him. With a twinkle in his eye, he had let me know that I should do what I wanted: I had his blessing, though writing wasn't for him.

In the spring of 2006 I was on an almost non-stop book tour. As often as my conscience allowed, I would leave my partner and spend the weekend in Wolfurt. I was a mess. Often I felt torn between love, family, and career. Sometimes one of them seemed burdensome, sometimes another. I was not used to such a nomadic lifestyle, nor to proper time management, and taking on responsibilities was not one of my strengths. I had always seen myself as a playful kind of guy, as someone who couldn't give up his route across the rooftops. Never mind. We always give our lives a form, and life always smashes it.

By the start of the summer of 2006 I finally had most of my author engagements behind me. I took my bike apart and packed it into my mother's car along with my bags. I drove to Wolfurt via Munich, arriving scarcely six hours later with a slight headache. It was the day before my father's eightieth birthday.

I slipped into some work clothes, whose smell betrayed how long they had lain around in an empty flat, jumped out of the window, and started picking wild strawberries and raspberries on the hillside below the house. Cherries, too. Then I unpacked my things. When I met my father early that evening, he remarked, 'Ah, so you thought you'd come and see if I was still alive.'

Physically, he was still in fine fettle. If you met him on the street, you wouldn't at first think that there was anything wrong with him. He smiled warmly at everyone and manoeuvred his way through short exchanges with little jokes, so that people claimed that he *always* recognised them and was the same old mischief-maker as ever. Only when the conversation touched on a topic that needed more context and understanding were his weaknesses revealed.

Now he would sit on the stone wall in front of the house, after first spreading out his handkerchief underneath him, and look down the quiet road. Patiently, he waited for something to happen. For what? He had modest needs. If a car drove by, he would wave. If a woman went past on a bicycle, he would say, 'Good afternoon, beautiful lady.'

Nothing to worry about.

The bells of the nearby church rang out on the hour. My mother went over to him. Seeing that he had some breadsticks poking out of the pocket of his left trouser leg, she suggested he remove them or else he would get crumbs in his pocket. He said, 'I need them for my morning shave.'

'You can't shave with them, August.'

He thought about that and replied, 'Later today, I'll put them in the soil in the garden, then they'll sprout and something beautiful will grow.'

That was rather more worrying.

He got up, and after he had picked up and folded his handkerchief with a reserved dignity, he walked around to the terrace behind the house. I followed him. We didn't say anything but looked west towards Lake Constance, where the sunset lingered as if the day didn't want to end. There were wispy clouds on the hill above St Gebhard's Church, blue sky everywhere else. We listened to the quiet murmur of the wind in the birch leaves and the distant thrum of the A14 highway in the Rhine Valley. The family orchard below us was a lush green. There were the fruit trees and the beehive, almost unchanged since he, and then I, had been a child.

'You'll be eighty tomorrow,' I said to him.

'Me?' he asked.

'Yes, you. You'll be eighty, Dad.'

'Not me,' he said, laughing with mock indignation. He looked at me and added, 'You, perhaps.'

'I'll be thirty-eight, Dad, but tomorrow you'll be eighty.'

'Not me,' he repeated, amused. 'You, perhaps.'

It went back and forth like this for a while, until I asked him how it felt to be eighty. Then he said, 'You know, I can't claim it's anything special.'

Two hours later, after I had picked some more raspberries, I put him to bed and finally let the rudder drift, falling into bed in a stupor, exhausted from the previous weeks of touring and the long drive.

Early in the morning I wished my father a happy birthday, which he accepted willingly enough, thanking me. As he sat on the edge of the bed in his underpants, I made the observation that at the age of eighty, his father hadn't been alive any more. He looked at me in surprise and then smiled weakly. But I couldn't tell what his smile meant. When I said that we were going to celebrate his birthday in the church hall, he wanted to know which one.

'The Wolfurt church hall,' I said.

'I've always liked visiting Wolfurt. I get along well with everyone.'

*

The day went smoothly. It was a Tuesday and the party was planned for Friday. I remember that my mother had baked a fruit flan and that a neighbour brought over a little birthday card, remarking to us that the lane wouldn't be half as beautiful without August's smile. That delighted me, because at that point I wasn't yet aware that his character was largely intact. Back then I believed that the illness was destroying his personality.

Helga and Werner came in the evening. We all ate cake and drank wine, and Werner and I watched a World Cup semi-final. Our father sat with us but the game – between Germany and Italy – made little impression on him, because it was tactical without any obvious climaxes. Our father kept asking, 'So who's playing? Wolfurt and who else?'

'Kennelbach,' I kept replying.

He nodded, as if he should have figured it out by himself, and said in annoyance, 'They always play like that!'

When Fabio Grosso scored the first goal, he said, 'Hold on. That's not Wolfurt.'

Werner and I split our sides laughing. And those moments were the highlights of the game for us. If it weren't for them, we wouldn't remember it now.

*

I remember his fiftieth birthday equally well. I was eight. Werner and I shared a bedroom, and from one of its windows we peered excitedly at the party guests on the terrace. It was also the day on which our father, after almost thirty years, stopped smoking.

Fireworks shot into the sky over Bregenz, because 4 July 1976 was also the two hundredth anniversary of American independence. With their rockets, the Americans put an extra glow on the day, and to us children it reflected on our father.

His younger colleagues dived out of the window into the swimming pool.

*

At his eightieth birthday party he bade 'All the best, health and happiness' to everyone in the long line of well-wishers, clasping their hands with both of his own. He appeared to be full of life, was obviously enjoying the event, and didn't look like someone simply resigned to carrying out his birthday duties. My father told the mayor, whom he had trained during his last year at the parish offices, not to talk so much but to sing something instead. He got some laughs for that.

My brothers and sister had prepared a little Power-Point presentation with photos from his long life. I was sitting at the table with many of our father's siblings, so I couldn't see the impression the pictures made on him. He was no doubt swept up in the excitement as the guests went *ah* and *oh* and laughed. It was only when an image appeared of his grandfather, the smith, in a long leather apron and with a heavy hammer resting on his shoulder, that my father started to talk about his failings as usual. 'I'm of no use to anyone now – damn it – never mind – it's hardly earth-shattering news.'

Family photos from the early fifties glowed on the white wall: Adolf and Theresia Geiger, surrounded by the nine children who still lived at home at that time, just a little before Emma, one of the three daughters, died of a ruptured appendix. It was astonishing how old the grandparents looked, even back then. They seemed to be about to enter their dotage, although my grandmother would go on to live another forty years, outwardly almost unchanged, a small worn-out woman with grey hair and deep lines in her face.

Apart from one son, all the surviving members of the family had come – they were people from a different era, farm children who had sharpened their slate pencils on the cellar step because it was made of sandstone and was particularly good for whetting. Our odd clan had proven itself absurdly inventive and capable, with an imagination that had a practical rather than a visionary bent. Only Josef was missing. He was the only one who had pulled away from the family's magnetic field. He emigrated to the United States in the late fifties and made his American Dream happen by inventing an electric can opener.

I asked the brothers and sisters if one of them, by any chance, had a copy of the photo of my father taken soon after he was released from the POW camp. They all knew immediately which photo I meant, but simultaneously shook their now-grey heads. Maria, over eighty years old, said that it was different back then, when you couldn't make as many copies of a photo as you wanted.

Paul told us about his own homecoming and how he had been confronted with a devastating image. Not long before his return, a thunderstorm had blown through the orchard – trees were flat on the ground and weeds covered everything. Most men of working age were away because of the war, and the women had their hands full with the livestock and housework. Robert, who was nine when the war ended, said he had been working in the field when the storm took him by surprise, and that he had held on to a tree trunk while the hail beat down on his legs. The cartload of hay, which the children were rushing to bring inside, almost tipped over near the limekiln. And because the hail had destroyed the fruit, many of the trees started to flower in the autumn.

My father had forgotten all of that; it no longer pained him. He had transformed memories into character, and his character remained. His formative experiences were still at work.

*

That year, like every summer, I spent some weeks at my parents' house. I could feel that the distance that had grown between my father and me was now closing again, and that we weren't losing touch, which is what I had long feared from the illness. Instead, there was an uncomplicated warmth between us, thanks to his forgetfulness, so that I almost welcomed this failing. All our conflicts were in the past. 'An opportunity like this won't come around again,' I thought.

My partner Katharina, who at the time lived in Innsbruck, came to spend a few days in Wolfurt. One day we persuaded my father to go for a walk with us. He came along reluctantly and kept wanting to turn back, although we hadn't yet left the upper field. I was a little exasperated, because it was a beautiful evening and I would have liked to walk down to the river with him.

When we turned into the lane by the house and the view down to Wolfurt unfolded in front of us, he was happy and praised the panorama.

'Have you often walked here?' he asked me. 'Some people come just for the view.'

That sounded odd to me, and I replied, 'I don't come here because of the view. I grew up here.'

That seemed to surprise him. He made a face and muttered, 'Oh, right.'

So I asked, 'Dad, do you know who I am?'

The question seemed to embarrass him. He turned to Katharina and, waving vaguely in my direction, joked, 'As if that were really so interesting.'

Dad, what was the happiest time of your life?

When they were young.

Who are you talking about? When who was young?

Oh, my kids.

The undermining of religious and bourgeois conventions during the Nazi era led indirectly to these same conventions being held in exaggerated esteem after the war. Paul told me that the social landscape after the war was as bleak as the moon's surface: piety, conservatism, a sense of decency, and nothing but work. For young people it was ghastly, he said.

Given my father's modest dreams, he couldn't have found the situation quite so claustrophobic. He was more interested in avoiding pain than in seeking out happiness. Back in Wolfurt, he could live the life he believed was right and at the same time regain a sense of security and stability. He wanted no more surprises, which also meant no more opportunities. To be open to the opportunities the world offers you, you need trust, and trust – if my father had possessed it before the war – had been taken from him. Experience forms scar tissue.

His need for a quiet life steered him to work for local government and to help in village associations. He was one of the founding members of the local football team and played as a winger. He led the amateur dramatics society and directed Nestroy's *Lumpazivagabundus*. He sang in the church choir, which was mainly made up of women. But women were rather exotic objects to him and in them he showed no interest. For the post-war decade, there were no skirts in his life, except for his mother's.

Maybe he had no need to prove his masculinity, maybe he valued his independence. A kiss in those days meant something different to a girl than it does today.

After a few years' work as the fuel management specialist for Vorarlberg's government, he became the clerk for Wolfurt in 1952 (or, in German, the *Gemeindeschreiber*, literally the 'parish writer'), and indeed, until the mid-1960s, he had no secretary to help him. My father's office was in a former classroom on the ground floor of the village school. It was an enormous space, much too big; the furniture was ancient and there were no curtains. In the summer he would sit there in his lederhosen and sandals, typing away, with two fingers pounding on the typewriter keys and the sound echoing around the large empty room. When he had the window open, his typing could be heard from the street, and people would say, 'August's clattering away again.'

There was a teacher who came to Vorarlberg from the easternmost state of Burgenland. Her name was 'Terusch', and my father apparently liked her. But Dätt was against her for some reason or other, and my father followed his father's will. The story is a little vague and I haven't been able to verify anything; my father's siblings know nothing about it and I can't ask him myself.

I do know that at that time, at the end of the fifties, my father started to build a house on the hillside above his parents' orchard. Dätt had been happy to give him the land 'because the grass doesn't grow up there.' From then on, my father spent his free hours on the building site. It wasn't far from the church, and the leaden vibrations of the tolling bell would often ring through the air.

In *The Dominion of the Dead*, Robert Pogue Harrison writes that according to an ancient strain in Western philosophy, you must know something before you can make it. If you want to build a house, you have to know what a house is before you start. My father *sort of* knew. He knew the basics. He planned everything himself, he made his own hollow bricks, he did the electrics himself, and did the plastering himself. He liked plastering, he said. He felt 'at home' with things like that.

The new house stood above the orchard with the nobility of something freshly made and freshly whitewashed. To the left were the Swiss mountains and Appenzell, then Wolfurt and Bregenz straight ahead, and to the right the Gebhardsberg and the sheer cliffs of the Känzele. The view lent a special charm to the location. Many years later, when I asked my father why the house stood as it did, he replied that he hadn't positioned it according to the sun, but the Gebhardsberg.

*

In 1963, at the age of thirty-seven, my father ended up marrying after all. He walked down the aisle with a young teacher from St Pölten, who – by his standards – hadn't had a home. Her father, a locomotive stoker, fell in the war. She grew up in terrible poverty. Her mother worked in a children's home in Ybbs and mended people's clothing on the side. The daughter, after her mother remarried, was sent to stay with her grandfather in Vorarlberg, where she trained as a teacher. Her first posting was the old schoolhouse in Wolfurt.

My mother had gone from the province to the depths of the province. And it was there she made a mistake, she would later tell me.

Those short of sense when they marry pay dearly to acquire it later. Such a practical attitude to marriage was light years away from my parents' approach. Because they hadn't been shown by example in their childhood homes, their ideas were based largely on ignorance – and, as is so often the case, on failing to see that they couldn't change the other person. Character is a harder currency than good will.

Unsuited as they were for each other, they had made a spectacular mistake. I can't put it any better than Tolstoy, who wrote in *Anna Karenina* that allowing young people to choose their spouse is about as sensible as suggesting that loaded pistols are an appropriate toy for five-year-olds, as the old princess says.

Before the wedding, it didn't occur to my parents to think what would happen when their two different ideas of happiness clashed. Both of them were capable of being happy, but examined more closely, it was clear that they had very different ways of reaching that happiness. In the end, they were each unhappy in their own way.

Neither could meet the other's expectations. They even communicated in essentially different ways. Their ages and backgrounds left an unbridgeable chasm between them: my father was from a large farming family, my mother from a single-parent, working-class home; he had been socialised in the pre-war years, she post-war; the war and imprisonment were formative for him, poverty and the *Heimatfilm* genre for her. Different expectations, different values, different emotional tones: he favoured the simple and bare, she favoured the sensual and warm; he was fond of company, she loved education. He often gave her proof that he wasn't cut out for a more cultured life. She would tell us, 'August fell asleep in the first act.'

Their separate dreams created a perfect dissonance, excepting the wish to marry and have children. Apart from those shared goals, their daily life together resembled that of two people in the Tower of Babel, desperately insisting, each in their own language, 'You don't understand me!'

When I asked my father why he had married my mother, he said that he had liked her a lot and wanted to give her a home. Here, too, his great themes were present: home, safety, security. They were what mattered to him. Being in love is nice, he might have thought, but knowing where you belong is nicer still.

Meanwhile, my mother wasn't looking for safety and security, but for stimulation. She was open to the world and hungry for what was *new*. There was no question of a honeymoon, because they had no money. But when my father refused to go on a walk and call it their honeymoon, my mother was flabbergasted. To my father, the only point of the world being so large and beautiful was so that everyone didn't crowd into Wolfurt.

'Not even a walk in the woods!' my mother would often recount with indignation. His refusal was certainly not his finest hour. My father didn't want his habits disturbed for a single day. Anything that broke the routine was unwelcome, even a little excursion on the Saturday afternoon after his wedding.

His life plan: no winding lines, just straight ones.

*

Writing about a failed marriage seems a little like sweeping up cold ashes. For a time the two of them must have managed, by compromising, to negotiate some approximation of inner peace. They didn't argue, and in spite of the tensions in their relationship, the birth of their children brought some equilibrium. As one baby followed another in quick succession, my mother was very happy, while my father's efforts to be a good husband meant striving to do well in his role as a father – and he did. The happiness of having children was something my parents could share. But as a relationship based on love, the marriage was a hopeless failure. The utterly different nature of their feelings played one trick after another on them and they gradually became more intransigent in their attitudes. When two people have such completely opposed ways of thinking, at some point they will come to the conclusion that further debate and concessions have no point.

Early in their marriage, life in the large house on the hill followed a more or less normal course. We looked like a normal family. We played our musical instruments for hours each day, and after lunch those children who could already hold cards would play canasta for half an hour with our parents. Before lunch, we children ran down to the church square to wait for our father, who came home from the office for two hours each afternoon. At that hour, the whole village seemed peaceful and friendly, with the smell of food wafting through the gardens and streets, because almost every household would sit down to eat at twelve on the dot. My father would put one of us children on his bike rack, one on the handlebars, all the rest of us would run alongside. On Saturday afternoons he took us with him to the football fields, and on Sundays we went on excursions. My father tended a vegetable patch with strawberries, too, and he also made lemon-balm cordial and elderberry juice. And when our mother said it was impossible to keep an eye on all four of her children at the lake, and that my father would have to go with them next time, he built a swimming pool. At first he had hatched a daring scheme to put the pool on the roof of the garage, connecting it to the balcony via a rope bridge. Such ideas were never lacking.

In spite of the difference in my parents' ages, my father made no pretence about being the head of the family. He was happy when he was left in peace. There was nothing strict about him. Yet he didn't help with housework, although his wife was soon working again. He firmly believed that there was man's work and woman's work, ordained by right and by God. Tidying up was for women, except in the garden; hammering was for men, except when preparing schnitzel.

The house was always a construction site, with no end to the extensions and renovations. My father never stopped thinking about possible improvements to the house or garden. In this respect, you could ask anything of him. Another bedroom? It couldn't hurt. And so we would have more room inside and he would have something else to plaster.

Driven by her longing for 'the world', my mother started to rent out rooms in the summer. She preferred German and Dutch travellers who were looking for a handy spot halfway between Lake Constance and the Bregenz Forest. After my father had converted the attic into a bedroom, they took in lodgers all year round – my mother's teaching colleagues and young people who didn't expect anything too fancy.

In 1977 'the world' really did come to my mother. We had a lodger from Germany whose surname was

Pech – which in German means 'bad luck', but also the tarry waterproofing substance 'pitch'. And the name fit: he had dark hair and liked to wear black. No one knew exactly what his job was, but he was warm-hearted and nice, and bought Ovaltine, which we children ate straight from the tin. When we were supposed to bring old magazines to the church youth group and everyone else came with the weekly television guides and church newspapers, I once took copies of *Stern* and *Der Spiegel* that Pech would regularly throw on the recycling pile under the stairs – and was immediately sent home with 'that stuff'. One evening Pech came down from the attic and said he had to leave, that he didn't have money to pay his last instalment of rent, but he'd leave his radio and hotplate. My father agreed, and the lodger moved out. A few days later, the police knocked on the door and asked after Pech, who was suspected of being a member of the militant Red Army Faction (RAF). We told them he'd gone.

At the same time the hosiery and lingerie manufacturer Walter Palmers was kidnapped by members of the militant 2 June Movement – and it was a Vorarlberger who had made the ransom demands over the telephone, clear from his accent. In an attempt to identify him, the newspaper printed a number you could call to hear the man's voice. I was nine at the time and secretly dialled the number several times. I found his words spooky and funny, although I had no idea what they meant. When it turned out that the Vorarlberger was a young man from Wolfurt, the general consternation reached its height.

My mother had taught him at school, she told us, and he had been a very nice quiet boy, she had liked him.

We didn't hear from Pech for many years. We children were pleased to have harboured a wanted terrorist and to have eaten up his Ovaltine. We thought Wolfurt was the secret centre of the RAF. And then one day, Pech was there on our doorstep, just dropping by. We felt a little awkward as our father told him about the police investigation, but Pech waved it away. They had found him quickly and just as quickly let him go again – all part of the hysteria of 1977.

Our father was visibly relieved, and I, a little disappointed.

My childhood was reaching its end. My father had been a good and happy father until then – the time when he should have taken more initiative. He wasn't comfortable with adolescents, which is common enough among parents. He should have been trying to interest his children in new things, but it wasn't in his nature to reach out to people. He preferred to withdraw and settle deeper into the old habits of his village life. The words 'habit' and 'inhabit' are related, of course.

When the phone rang, our father didn't make a move to get it. He couldn't imagine that anyone would want anything of him.

'Won't be for me,' he would say.

Nor did he wait for the postman. Why would he? The postman never brought him anything worth looking forward to.

Increasingly, I saw my father as a person who had nothing in common with me. And as it wasn't possible to direct my youthful need for rebellion against my father's authority (since he never showed any desire to lord it over anyone), I took the alternative route and rebelled against my father's ignorance. Most people tend to find their parents' care is either excessive or lacking. I reproached him for not showing any interest, but my accusations didn't get a rise out of him, which annoyed me all the more. I couldn't understand his behaviour and so neither could I accept it. There came a time when I wrote him off as someone I no longer wanted to bother with. I had enough 'other problems'. That was true, but it was also a cop-out, because I had become interested in other things, as happens at that age. It got so bad that, to be honest, I wasn't hoping for a future where the gap between my father and me would close again. Back then my father wasn't particularly important to me; at times I ignored him completely.

As a teenager, I noticed that he wasn't quick or harsh in his judgements, and that he didn't like to speak ill or thoughtlessly of others. I valued that in him, from an ever greater distance.

He was now spending a lot of time in his cellar workshop. There, he was free to let his thoughts wander and dive into crazy schemes. There he could keep his life free of external events. His workshop was his refuge and his natural home. Even today I am amazed at how well he organised it. In the seventies he fixed a wide board to the low ceiling and nailed the lids of baby-food jars onto it, screw sides facing down. He filled the jars with the small items he had sorted, and dozens of jars hung from the ceiling, easy to take in at a glance – so perfectly ordered that even his wife and children could always find what they were looking for.

If someone asked, 'Where's Dad?' the answer was normally, 'Probably in his workshop.'

'What's he tinkering with?'

'Oh, something or other.'

*

My memories of the time are full of situations like that. We didn't want our father, who was pottering about on the edge of our family life, to disturb us in absentia: the electric drill in the cellar that blurred the television screen, the constant knocking and rapping from some corner or other when we children had homework to do or wanted to read. When my father got ill, my first thoughts followed the same pattern – I didn't want my father to withdraw due to his illness and by his absence affect me. In fact, he continued to live his autonomous Robinson Crusoe existence when he fell ill. His family was the background he needed – the sea and the wind and the forest and the goats and his Man Friday.

Robinson Crusoe is the only novel that our father read in his whole life, and he read it many times. It is one of the few masterpieces of world literature in which not love, but instead self-assertion, is the most important element. Our father christened his first car (a 1934 DKW convertible) 'Robinson'. He even drove that car down to South Tyrol for several days with friends. That was in 1955, the year he bought it, long before he married my mother.

*

The eighties were marching on. My parents had not exactly developed into paragons of domestic harmony. Time had brought out, rather than smoothed away, their differences. There was an ugly atmosphere at home, and their children's growing up hastened the disintegration. And because it's assumed that a family should be harmonious, soon each of us had the sense of being in the wrong. The time came when all of us felt isolated, left to our own devices and busy with our own affairs, which were of no concern to anyone else.

Uncle Josef once said, 'In our home a lot of things weren't right either. When we had a problem at school, we didn't even tell one of our brothers. And when we were happy about something, we kept it to ourselves – we went to our rooms and leapt up and down.'

When I was a teenager, I saw things that way too. I could only feel at home by blocking myself off from my family. Towards the end, we were all fed up with each other. At least it felt like that to me.

By the time I left high school, our family's breakdown was having a noticeable impact on everyone's states of mind. Thankfully, the process wasn't irreversible, as we learnt when the situation improved in later years. All of this has been wiped clean from my father's mind. For now, only my memory lingers.

During my school years I didn't always make life easy for my mother and father. My mother, too, was starting to find the boundaries of her existence constricting. When I think back, I'm no longer surprised that she was often in a bad mood. We arrived at my school-leavers' ball after an argument at home, and at the event my mother remained annoyed, because of all my schoolmates, I was the only one not wearing a collared shirt. My father took me aside to talk about it with me in his calm way, asking how I would feel if he bought a shirt from one of the waiters. To show me that he was serious, he took his wallet (with the photo) out of the inner pocket of his jacket. I could see that he had enough money with him. He told me that that every waiter kept a spare shirt in case they spilt something, and I should think about it – it wouldn't hurt to do it. I looked at him as if he were from another planet and refused, saying that I didn't want to stand there in the waiter's shirt. Looking back, I can see that his suggestion was made in good faith, and that he was trying to keep the peace.

*

A few weeks later I left Wolfurt and headed off to university.

What's the most important thing in life to you, Dad?

I don't know. I've experienced a lot of things. But . . . 'important'?

Does anything spring to mind?

It's important that people around you talk in a friendly way. Then most things are fine.

What don't you like as much?

When I have to obey. I don't like being hurried here and there.

Who hurries you?

Right now – nobody.

On cold or rainy days at the end of the seventies, we sat at the kitchen table and played The Game of Life, a harmless enough board game about financial success, suitable for children aged ten and up. The brightly illustrated board led you through all of life's stages. You spun a wheel and took whatever the wheel dictated: education, travels, marriage, success, a lack of success, houses that were built, houses that burned down again, setbacks in your career, an oil strike, bad investments, your silver wedding anniversary, retirement. We were unaware at the time that the route around the board was a piece of cake compared to what was actually ahead of us. And we had no idea that it really is often a matter of luck whether you fall back or get ahead.

When someone had an accident or missed a turn because of an illness, we laughed with glee.

*

My father's spatial orientation was deteriorating. At night he would wander around the village in his pyjamas. We were worried he'd have an accident. To make sure someone could keep an eye on him at night too, we decided on a twenty-four-hour care shift schedule. The door to the staircase was locked at night.

The Slovakian women who came to the house brought order to our father's daily routine. The constant stream of new faces entering his bedroom each morning had left him confused. Now his morale improved and we could see his vitality returning. This change, and the fact that as the illness progressed its impact was milder, allowed our father to enter a relatively good period. No two people affected by dementia are alike, and any generalisations are problematic. Those affected by the illness remain essentially unfathomable, each one of them a particular case with his or her own abilities and feelings, in whom dementia takes a different course. In my father's case, it progressed slowly, and the less he was aware of his wretched condition, the less the disease affected his mood. Although he was fully aware of the dementia, it no longer scared him. Calmly, he accepted his fate, and his underlying positive attitude was once again visible.

He now seldom wandered around the house looking for a port in a storm. There were still situations in which he wanted to go home, but the wish was no longer accompanied by panic. His voice often sounded peaceful, like the voice of someone who knows life always ends badly and that there's no point in getting worked up about it.

'I'm going home now,' he said once, when he was tired of waiting any longer for someone to take him. 'Are you coming with me or staying here?'

'I'll stay here.'

'OK, then I'm going on my own. Why would I wait here and then, perhaps, go home in November? And maybe have to pay something, too. My only chance is to go now.'

'Yes, you might as well go.'

'Can I go?'

'If you want to. No one's stopping you.'

'And one more thing, my family – can I take them, too?'

'Of course. Take them too.'

'Good. Thank you.'

He looked around to see if he could think of anything else he ought to take, and, satisfied there wasn't, said, 'Nothing here affects me personally.'

Then he came over to the table again. I could see from the expression on his face that he found something a little embarrassing. He hesitated, but in the end came out with what was bothering him.

'Could you give me the address? Or directions? I mean, you just have to tell me, "Go up the street until you see the house."'

The manner in which he asked for my help touched me deeply. I said, 'I've thought about it – I'll go with you. If you can wait half an hour, until I've finished typing, we'll go together.'

'Where?' he asked.

'Home,' I said. 'I feel like going home, too.'

'Really?'

'Really. But before we go, you should rest a bit and gather your strength.'

'Is it far?'

'Far enough. But we can walk it.'

'And you really would come too?'

'Yes, of course.'

'You'd do that?'

I took his hand and squeezed it briefly. 'More than happy to.'

He liked that answer. A smile immediately lit up his whole face, and, grasping my hand, he exclaimed, 'Thank you!'

Then he sat down at the table and we had a fairly peaceful evening until his carer put him to bed.

*

At this time, he mostly thought I was his brother Paul. I didn't care – at least it was family. Nor did I mind when he greeted me in the morning with a sing-song, 'Hello-o, dear bro-o-ther.'

Sometimes he swapped over mid-sentence. He introduced me once as his brother Paul, 'the forester', before adding, 'He's a poet and thinker.'

He almost never ran away any more. He liked to sit on the little wall in front of the house or stand on the terrace and look at the village below. I sometimes expected that he, as if healthy again, was going to turn to me and start a casual conversation. We'd never had anything other than casual conversations. He'd never had a serious discussion with me, never given me advice. I can't remember any fatherly chats. His MO was to comment on the weather or the shifts in the landscape.

When you saw him in the dappled shade of one of the trees, you might think everything was fine.

Back then, I thought the time remaining was short. I wondered where we would be next year, or the year after. Two or three years – that's about the time I take to write a novel. Three years, the length of time that I believed I would be able to reach my father. So I came to Vorarlberg as often as I could and gave his carers afternoons off, so I could spend time alone with him.

Most days went very peacefully. Sometimes I thought there was something wrong with my ears, because I wasn't used to the silence. As I worked, my father sat opposite me at the kitchen table. He slid his hands back and forth over its surface, sometimes took rapid and rhythmical breaths, or fiddled with the newspaper rack, but mostly he was calm. Sometimes he asked a question and we talked, and sometimes he peered over at my laptop screen and read along. When I asked him if he was interested in what I was writing, he said, 'Yes, I'm allowed some interest.'

Then he sat down again and his face went blank, as if he were dreaming. His absent-mindedness made me feel he was his old self again. He played with his fingers as if there were nothing more urgent at that moment, occasionally asking me to let him know, should I need any help. 'Unfortunately,' he added, 'I know I don't get good results any more. My performance is weak. It's difficult. I won't be able to help you much.'

I said, 'Of everyone, you help me the most.'

'Don't say that!' he replied.

'But it's true, you help me the most.'

'It's nice of you to say so.'

'It's true.'

He brooded over that for a moment before saying, 'Then for now, I'll take note of that.'

When he sat alone in the living room, he often sang, and more and more often he would really belt it out. I thought that if he continued like that he'd make it to ninety. He led a healthy life, after all. Every day he had regular meals, sang, went for walks and slept long. There was no meat on Fridays: his Slovakian carers held to that. And on Sundays they would accompany him to church, if Peter and his family had already gone the previous evening.

*

When he sang, he would change the words for fun. In speech, too, he became more inventive again. His former mischievousness returned, like the beauty you see when an overgrown garden has been thinned out a little.

'I also took part in those things,' he said. 'But please don't mistake that "part" for something big – I think small.'

I was impressed by how he expressed himself, I felt in contact with words' magic potential. James Joyce claimed that he had no imagination but simply accepted what language offered him. It seemed the same with my father. From the German word *zukünftig* ('of the future'), he switched letters to make *kuhzünftig* ('of the cows' guild'). When I announced that I was stumped, which in German is to be 'at the end of my Latin', *am Ende des Lateins*, he again switched letters, saying he himself wasn't so much *am Ende des Lateins* as *am Ende des Duseíns* ('at the end of his existence'), stressing the words in a way that emphasised his pun. And some old phrases that I hadn't heard for a long time came back:

'You can't make the sheet bigger by pulling at it.'

'A good stumbler won't fall.'

'You act as if you had shoe nails in your soup.'

When he couldn't think of a word, he would say, 'I don't know how I should christen it.'

Words popped easily out of his mouth. He was relaxed and said what he thought, and what he thought was often not only original but had hidden depths. *Why don't I think like that!* I was amazed at how precisely he expressed himself, how he would get the tone just right, how skilfully he chose his words. 'You and I,' he said, 'We're going to make life as nice as possible for each other, and if that doesn't work out, one of us will be left standing.'

At such times it was as if he were stepping out of the house of his illness to enjoy the fresh air. For short periods he was once again himself. We had some lovely hours, all the more special because they were wrestled from the illness.

'My assessment is that I'm doing well,' he said. 'I'm now an old man. Now I have to do what I like doing and see how things turn out.'

'And what do you want to do, Dad?'

'Nothing, actually. That's the beauty of it, you know. It takes skill.'

*

Even when blood in his urine proved to be the result of a bladder tumour, he didn't seem put out. He remained cheerful and was just a little 'surprised'. Only after the operation was he out of sorts, because of the anaesthetic and the strange environment. Everyone was happy when the doctors finally discharged him. He quickly recovered and even knew that he was home. No small feat.

In the hospital, he had woken up and said to his carer, Daniela, that he was in pain. Daniela replied that she couldn't help him, but she would stay there with him. He then said, 'If you stay here with me, that's already a great help.'

My father was also diagnosed with type 2 diabetes, and every morning he showed a remarkable ability to swallow pills of any size without water, while making a comical, screwed-up face. He would only drink the water when the pill was already down.

For a while he hadn't been able to recognise the television as another reality. He asked how it was that when he looked over, there would be a room he didn't know one minute, and a car the next.

'How did the car get in here?'

This culminated one day around Christmas when he was watching the news on the sofa. He got up and offered the newsreader the tray of Christmas biscuits, encouraging him to take one. When the man didn't respond, our father took one of the jam biscuits, and, holding it up to the spot where the newsreader's mouth was moving, suggested he try it. The man's continued rudeness irritated our father. The scene, in spite of its comedic value, scared us. It was eerie.

The illness was certainly bringing forth some outlandish fruit by this time. These strange episodes were normally short, and often they indicated that our father didn't feel his best. His condition could quickly alter, depending on whether or not he was in good hands.

Some of his carers were like dear friends to him; others didn't manage to make him feel safe and secure. Then he would get confused and scared, and would start to panic because he thought he was in real danger.

'They're shooting – take cover!' he shouted. 'It's the Swiss, shooting at us again!'

*

Grey, slightly brown smoke rose up from my grand-parents' house. Uncle Robert was making schnapps. That morning, Uncle Erich had been out in the field with a bucket and a small shovel, digging up the young oaks that had taken seed. The smoke from the chimney had become almost invisible – maybe it was the second stage of distillation. From my window I could see the walnut tree beyond the chimney shimmering a little in a haze.

It was a cool day with wisps of high clouds. A flock of finches was looking for food among the raspberry bushes.

I was working on the idea for my novel *All About Sally* and drinking coffee from a battered old cup when my mobile rang. It was Maria, one of the carers. She had wanted to give my father a shower, but he hadn't wanted one, and so he locked himself in the bathroom the moment she left the room. Now he wasn't coming out.

I went upstairs to help. I begged repeatedly before my father opened the door. He was sitting on the bathroom stool in his trousers and a white undershirt, his skin hanging slackly from his arms. The two towels around his neck were knotted together on his chest, and in one hand he held up a long-handled back scrubber, and in the other, nail clippers with the file flicked out. He did look like a king now, with a sceptre and sword. But his face bore the mark of madness.

I asked if he wanted to watch television with me.

He didn't look at me and his grim expression suggested he was determined to take things as far as possible. He was hallucinating. He kept looking into the shower and asking what he should do with 'the others'.

Since he was fumbling around with the giant brush and the file all this time, I was a little distracted. Instead of calming him down by letting him know I'd protect him and chase off 'the others', I tried to divert his attention – in vain. He still felt threatened. With his head hunched over, he kept darting glances left and right, alert to any dangers.

When I tried to take the scrubber from his hand, he made as if to hit me. I jumped back in surprise and then gave him an earful, shouting, 'Are you crazy? You're a pillar of the community – and that's how you behave?! Who taught you that? Certainly not your mother! And you never taught us, your children, to do anything of the sort!'

I really let it rip, mentioning all the things that would cut him to the quick. Interestingly, the lecture had an effect. He looked disconcerted, as if he were ashamed. Of his own initiative, he put down the scrubber and agreed when I said I was going to take the file. Now the worst was over. I helped him on with his shirt and steered him to the television. He appeared relaxed, exaggeratedly cheerful, and ready to joke around. Meanwhile, Maria was crying in her room. She had struggled with him for an hour and let him threaten her with the scrubber many times.

I called Helga, who was often first in the line of fire. Could she come and be there for Maria? I spent the evening with our father. The incident in the bathroom was the first time he had become aggressive. That night he was cheerful and made a special effort to be friendly, as if he knew that I was worried about him, and as if he were determined to make us forget his actions. This time the hellfire had only singed us.

But at that moment I couldn't see a way forward. Our father couldn't afford too many outbursts like this. His carers reacted badly to such escalations and he had even scared me – I'd had visions of a violent madman.

My father's sense of things might have been, *What does this woman want from me? That I shower? Just a trick! I'm not going to let strangers boss me around any longer. She barely speaks German and yet she thinks she has the right to order me around. Suspicious behaviour.*

He didn't like to remember the Soviet nurses from that ramshackle building near Bratislava. They had given him orders instead of care. Maybe something from those distant days had stuck and was now surfacing. No idea. In any case, it was a strange coincidence that his carers came to him in Wolfurt from Slovakia, and some were from Bratislava itself.

That evening we watched *Candid Camera* together. My father was interested, would laugh and comment on the 'nonsense', as he called it, while I typed up notes on my laptop about what had happened. I had given Maria the evening off, to recover. She missed home. A few days later, she quit.

Was it on that evening's *Candid Camera* that there was a scene in a hotel lift with the doors shut? Suddenly, the light went out, and when it went on again a few seconds later, a young man was missing. Only his bag was left on the floor. Most of the people in the lift reacted in shock, although one woman couldn't stop laughing hysterically.

When my father hallucinated, it must have felt similar in his head. Suddenly, the light would go out and he would be faced with a changed situation, with no explanation. A brain that has to constantly deal with such strange occurrences can't help but go into a state of alarm.

*

A few weeks later, Aunt Hedwig, Emil's wife, left a message on my answering machine. I called her back. It was about Katharina, my cousin Maria's daughter. A viral infection had left Katharina paralysed for weeks, and she was able to move only her eyes. Afterwards, she had recorded the whole experience, including the nightmares brought on by the medicine. Aunt Hedwig and I also talked about my father. She mentioned a trip that my cousin Stefan had gone on with him, during which my father had made a point of saying he'd always had it good in life. Aunt Hedwig was quite amazed at that. She heard so few people say anything like it. She commented that his attitude was all the more remarkable when you recalled the photo taken after his captivity.

I replied that it was a shame the photo had been lost along with his wallet. Aunt Hedwig said, 'Oh, Arno, we've got a copy. No idea how we came by it, but we've got one.'

'Are you sure?'

I described the photo.

'Yes, I'm sure. If you want, I'll dig it out for you. You can pick it up tomorrow.'

So I picked up the photo and made a copy of the copy and was allowed to keep the original copy. It's one of the things I treasure most.

The stamp on the back of the photo reveals that Emil made the copy in 1995, when he and my father were already old men. 1995. It was around then that the whole mess started.

*You know, I'm not such a young lad. You, on the other hand –
you're a spring chicken.*

True enough.

Some bits of me have got old.

But however old a person gets, he can always learn new things.

*Not me, sadly. There's nothing more in me. And I'd be very happy
if I could soon . . . soon . . . soon . . . not have to help out any
more. I'd prefer to take a stroll and do nothing.*

You can do nothing as much as you'd like.

*That's what you think. There's always something or other to be
angled into place. But I want to give that up soon.*

The water was gurgling down the drainpipe, a mesmerising and somewhat hostile sound. Against time and the weather we are powerless.

I mentioned the rain to my father. He looked over at the window and said, 'Oh, the beautiful times when I was young, when I was young, it was still beautiful outside. Now it's grim – grim.'

He hadn't completely lost his sense of time yet, but, as he put it, he had 'a screw loose'. Confusingly, the very thing he kept was an understanding that his abilities were waning. It was an increasingly common topic of his conversation, something I found all the more surprising, given the fact that he was no longer able to master everyday tasks. He didn't know if he was hungry or thirsty, and it was 'not an easy thing' to eat and drink in the usual way. Once, a slice of bread was on his plate and he apologised for not knowing what to do with it. He asked me for advice.

'Just take a bite,' I said.

Instruction didn't help. He answered sadly, 'Hmm. If only I knew how. You know, I'm a poor devil.'

He said he was a poor devil every few hours, but certainly not always in a sad tone or out of protest – normally in a friendly way, as if he had to make an important statement. 'I'm a person who has no say. Nothing to do about it now.'

Sentences like this could have come from a Kafka or Bernhard character, I thought – what a perfect pair, someone with Alzheimer's and a writer. In *Frost*, Thomas Bernhard's protagonist laments, 'But I'm utterly incapable, utterly incapable.' And at another point, 'Everything is incomprehensible to me / I don't understand anything / Nothing makes sense to me.'

'I don't understand all this!' my father kept saying, a comment on the opacity of the system into which he'd been dragged. And his follow-up sentence was categorical – 'I'm nothing now.'

Often my father went into detail in his evaluation of the situation. A shiver went down my spine at the calmness with which he made announcements about himself.

'I'm a nobody,' he said. 'Yes, yes, I was once upon a time. I started strongly. But now, I'm old . . . and with age came a certain lack of concern . . . no, not a lack of concern . . . that's a bad expression . . . problems arose.'

He made a sign for The End by crossing and uncrossing his hands in front of his stomach. Then he started to look in different drawers, opening and closing them. When I asked what he was looking for, he couldn't give me a concrete answer.

'Nothing. Nothing to pass on to someone or to work on.' He added a 'Yes, yes' and then said, 'I've seen things too, and in principle I'm happy I did. But I'm in no state for that any more.'

'And what state are you in, would you say, Dad?'

'A weak one. I can only achieve things with other people's help. Nothing much going on with me nowadays. Well, well, that's life, and I can't change it. A lot went wrong in my life, there's a lot – well, a lot could have gone better. But I don't mourn it. I have no complaints, although I haven't managed to do much lately. At first I still could, but then it got worse. I've had bad luck, too.'

'What bad luck did you have?'

'Something broke in my hands. Things weren't worth anything any more . . . not that I want to blame others. It was a loss of strength. I'm no longer fit for things. I haven't flourished in – let me see – months. Maybe even longer.'

'What were the times when you did flourish?'

'I don't dwell on them. I had good times. I was often happy. But . . . but . . . but . . . they're over now. Yes, some bits of me are broken, I know. But I don't need them any more.'

He went to the door and exclaimed, 'For God's sake!' Five seconds later, he sang a few bars of a song, then peered into the pots on the stove and went out into the gazebo. When he came back, I asked, 'And? What's new?'

'With me, nothing – there's nothing new with me. With you, always, and I'm happy about that. You know, nothing's going on with me. I'm weak, I achieve little, and that's how things turned out.' He sang a few more bars. 'Soon, I'll . . . lie flat.'

'What?'

'Do nothing. You know, I've got no important matters to hand. That's my feeling. I can't prove it, but my feeling is that I've got nothing important to hand. Yes, that's how it is. Whatever still has to be done, has to be done by other people.'

'No need to worry. I'll take care of things.'

He laughed and, taking my hand, said, 'Thanks, I just want to say thank you. I'm a poor devil. Once I was a – thanks for not making a fuss that nothing's going on with me.'

'Dad, everything's been done, everything is arranged. Now the sun's setting.'

'Do you think so?'

'I know it.'

'Thanks for telling me that. Unfortunately, I'm no good at anything any more.'

Then he sat down at the table and lowered his head onto his folded arms.

*

He was often worried that something might be left undone. When I came down from the attic one evening, I bumped into my father and his carer Ludmilla in the first-floor hallway. Ludmilla was trying to put him to bed, but he was concerned that not everything was done and that someone was waiting for him. I told him there would be nothing more today, and it was bedtime for everyone. Distressed, he asked, 'And who will dismiss the crew?'

I took his hand, and, squeezing it briefly, said, 'I'll dismiss them. They can go home now.'

Behind his doubt, a smile started to spread over his face. With a wink he said, 'You're my best friend!'

*

Everyday interactions with him were increasingly like fiction. We accepted all the faulty memories, paranoia and workarounds with which his mind defended itself against the hallucinations and everything else it didn't understand. The only remaining place where we could be together was the world as he understood it. We would say everything we could to affirm his sense of things and make him happy. We learnt that holding sanctimoniously to the truth was the worst approach of all. The truth didn't get us anywhere – it served no one well. To give someone with dementia an answer that, according to the usual rules, is objectively correct, but which pays no attention to the place where that person finds him- or herself, is to enforce a world that isn't his or her own.

So we struck out away from sober reality and would only return after long detours. When our father wanted to go home, I'd say, 'Let's see what I can do for you, I think I can help.' And when he asked after his mother,

I pretended to believe she was still alive and reassured him that she knew about everything and was taking care of him. He liked that. He would beam back at me and nod. His beaming and nodding were the return to reality.

Objective truth was often thrown under the bus. I didn't care – it was worthless. At the same time, I took more and more pleasure in letting my responses slide into fiction. There was only one standard in use: the more something soothed our father, the better.

In daily dealings with him, much was a question of technique. What was demanded of us was extremely complex. Terrible as it was for my father that his brain was deteriorating, for his relatives it was true that adversity sharpens the mind. Conversations with him were good mental exercises. They required a considerable amount of empathy and imagination. A good one managed, with the right words and the right gestures, to banish his unease for a while. As Felix Hartlaub once said in a different situation, 'Only officially recognised tightrope walkers can survive here.'

Daniela said that putting my father to bed and getting him up in the morning wasn't as difficult when she asked him questions.

'Are you tired?'

'Yes.'

'Would you like to go to bed?'

'Yes.'

You had to try to get him to express the desired wish through your questions. In this way you could bring some order to his disordered world. Commands, on the other hand, didn't work. If she said, 'August, you have to go to bed now,' then he would ask, 'Why?'

Once, when Daniela was ironing, my father lost patience and said he was going home – no question about it, he wasn't going to stand for it any more. Daniela looked at him in shock and said, 'August, you can't leave me here on my own! What will I do without you? If you go, I'm coming, too. But I just need to do the ironing first.'

He saw the point of that, and she said thanks. Daniela told us she always said thanks, even when she had just done something for him. It built him up, left him contented, and created a certain dependence. He would look for her all day, following her around the house. He needed a sense of security. Then he felt good. He knew that he needed someone if he were not to drown. Once he told her, 'I live in this house that I built all on my own. None of my family are here right now – I'm alone with my carers.'

Once when he asked me who was in the house besides him and me, and I told him that no one was, and we were alone right then, he found the answer unnerving. He said, 'That's no good. I need care. I'm in trouble without care.'

Such statements always shook me, because I never expected such a clear-eyed appraisal of the situation from him. I quickly said, 'I'm here. I can care for you.'

His expression brightened up and he replied, 'I think highly of you for that, for taking the time.'

On another day he said, 'No one has ever done any-thing for me. You, perhaps?'

'Yes, I have. Sometimes.'

Bitterly, he retorted, 'You've never done anything for me!'

*

Of all the carers, Daniela got along best with him. I could only shake my head in amazement at how well. I came up to them once when she was showing him photos of her husband. My father said he knew the man. Impos-sible, she replied, her husband lived in Slovakia. My father replied, 'I like you, even though I don't believe what you're telling me.'

She insisted that her husband had never visited Vorarlberg and that he couldn't speak a single word of German. 'Not a single word!' she repeated, to which my father said, 'You're a nice woman. There's nothing more I can add.'

Daniela said that her time with my father wasn't difficult. She said you just needed patience. If he didn't want to get up, she waited for him – she had time. And if he didn't want to shave, she said it didn't matter. Half an hour later, he'd normally forgotten that he'd just refused her. Each day she could wait as long as need be, twenty-four hours if necessary.

Most of the other carers didn't fare as well. When he refused to do something, they would get nervous.

Finely attuned to their nervousness, he would then be unable to appreciate their attention. Discouraged by such incidents, the mutual unease would ratchet up so high that, although our family gave extra support in such moments, there were more and more days where we were all ready for a straitjacket by the evening. Sometimes, standing under the shower, I had the feeling that I was still running. Once, when I passed the wardrobe, I felt a need to sit inside it. At night, staring from hot and sleepless eyes into the uncertain future of the next day, I recalled the Latin expression *nox est perpetua*. Night never ends.

*

Now and then, something like hope returned. But the lulls between outbursts became shorter and shorter. There was nothing we could do to change that. In an unpredictable atmosphere, the tension was sometimes hard to bear. It was terrible to see so much suffering on every side. The dysfunctional relationships between our father and some of his carers only fed the illness. The carers quickly reached their limits, which in turn had a negative effect on our father. The downward spiral continued.

It started early in the morning. You just couldn't please him. The first thing my father would say would be something like, 'If you knew how they mistreat me here . . .'

That was the tone he maintained all day. The music they played was something he had to endure. Lunch wasn't right for him. 'I don't think I'll eat it.'

Once, he went out into the garden after the meal and peed into the pot containing Werner's biggest cactus. I heard a splashing and rushed out, shouting, 'You can't do that!' His reply? 'Of course I can. That's the punishment for what they're doing to me. They deserve much worse.'

Worst of all were the nights when he woke and began to look for his children. This happened with surprising and inexplicable regularity. On these nights our father was inconsolable, miserable, despairing. It was as if it were wartime and he were wandering around between bombed houses, looking for a sign of life. Sometimes you could calm him down by saying that his children were coming in the morning. Sometimes he would search half the night, until he fell asleep in exhaustion. The next day he'd start searching again for his four little children who weren't lying in their beds, who weren't hiding under them either, nor were they giggling in the wardrobes behind the shirts. Our father was distraught that he couldn't find any of them.

'They've been taken away,' he would say. 'No one has seen them. I've looked for them for ages and have contacted all kinds of offices to get help finding them. Now I've lost all hope of seeing them again.'

When I said I believed they were safe, that they would marry and have their own children, he replied, 'Everything you say could be true. But I don't believe it.'

He knitted his brows as if trying to recall something, then pointed to the cupboard and suggested that must be the direction the children had been taken. 'And where to? They're gone – not here – they're gone – not here.'

It would have worked out well with Vlasta, but then Vlasta's mother fell ill and told her on the phone that it wasn't right that Vlasta was looking after strangers in Austria while her own mother lay in bed at home.

Although Anna was very clever and did her best, she didn't click with our father. It was like we were jinxed. When they went out walking and people asked my father who was with him, he'd say she was a silly cow who always got on his nerves.

One time – the worst case of all – he made a gesture as if to slit her throat. She was afraid he might go to a drawer and get out a knife. I hid my worry and said that she shouldn't take it seriously. But could I be sure? So I added, 'He's ill, so there's no harm in taking care. In the worst case scenario, he's neither particularly strong nor quick.'

Very reassuring.

The crazy thing was that as soon as one of the carers who didn't get along with him had left, and Daniela or my mother was on duty again, after two or three days my father was as peaceful as a lamb – cheerful, calm, outgoing, and as friendly as could be. Then we'd start to hear his oddball comments again.

'Are you content, August?'

'I'm always content. Even as a baby, I was content.'

I don't know how to go on.

I'll take care of everything.

You mustn't forget me. That would be unfair.

We won't do that.

But, you know, it's not all that easy!

There's no way we would forget you. Definitely not.

My father had been struggling with Alzheimer's for over a decade now. MRI cross-sections of his brain showed the extent of the destruction. And yet he stepped out of the illness for short periods almost every day, asking in different ways what was wrong with his head. He smacked his forehead. 'Something's not right there. Can you tell me how to fix it?'

Then he looked beseechingly at me and was disappointed when I answered, without conviction, 'Help is coming from Bregenz.'

That was what Kafka wrote in his diary on 6 July 1916, almost ten years to the day before my father's birth. Kafka continued in his entry, 'And when the sick man's eyes narrowed in doubt, the doctor added: "Bregenz in Vorarlberg." "That's far away," said the sick man.'

For my father, too, Bregenz was far away – at least, in the sense that he had little hope. In his lucid moments he yearned for a functioning brain, but his brain didn't get better. Banging his fist against his head didn't have the same effect as when, in my childhood, he stood up and banged on the television because the image had started to drift.

One cold spring day in 2009 Daniela was getting him ready for a walk. He already had his shoes and coat on. Daniela put his hat on his head and said, 'There's your hat.'

'That's all well and fine, but where's my brain?'

'Your brain is under your hat,' I said from the kitchen.

My father took off his hat, looked inside and replied, 'Now, that would be something.' He hesitated, thought about it and, putting his hat back on his head, asked shyly, 'Is it really under the hat?'

'Yes, it's where it should be,' I said.

He raised his eyebrows and, confused, followed Daniela to the door.

Such surreal moments became more frequent. They make for good stories – comic and a little bizarre. But if you listen carefully, besides the comedy, which is liberating, you hear anxiety and despair. And more and more often, it wasn't funny at all.

Many things were difficult because our father didn't understand the point of them. He would get angry because he had to take medicine that tasted bad. He didn't know that he would be worse off without the medicine. So he snapped, 'You can't do this to me!'

'It's for your own good.'

'Anyone can say that!' he replied curtly. 'Don't think I'll fall for an impostor like you. I know what dirty tricks you get up to.'

Of course I was aware that it was his illness talking. And yet finding oneself shouted at with no reason left a bitter feeling – and it was all the more bitter for people who had little experience of the illness and neither knew our father well nor had any familial obligation to him.

'Go away! If you don't let me be, I'll get a gun and blast your arse off!'

He said that to me. It made me laugh. It reminded me of how, as a child, I had threatened people with my big brother. But some of the carers found it hard not to read more into his exclamations than a simple message: in a world of unknown faces, he wanted to be left alone.

Daniela was with us for almost three years. Right to the end, she swore that she wouldn't easily find a job that she loved as much. To her, our father was ill, but also an intelligent man who was always ready to have fun. Yes, his brain sometimes played tricks on him, but she had known him long enough to know that he was really a harmless poor devil.

Every three weeks she went back home to Slovakia and someone else stood in for her. Unfortunately, for over two years, none of her colleagues managed to get along with our father nearly as well. As these carers only stayed for short periods, the difficulties they faced were understandable.

All too often our father was negative and challenging for them, from morning to night. He tended to reject people whom he didn't know and who confused him. Most of his carers talked too much to him and in the wrong tone, as if talking to a child. And because he was still an imposing person, with a broad forehead and expressive face, he intimidated them. Sometimes, when he felt cornered, he would push them away.

It did no good to assure them our father was actually a nice man, nor to advise them to stay out of his way when he was in a bad mood. That's easy to say. The carers weren't trained nurses, and not every person has, by nature, the skills needed to deal with people who have dementia. Eva, our father's youngest granddaughter, did. She had only known her grandfather with Alzheimer's, and the affection she had for him was so genuine that of course he responded. Because she was free in her attitude, her grandfather could be free in her presence too.

The same was true for Daniela. Right from the start she had got along well with him. She was perfectly relaxed around him and he seemed to be almost a little in love with her. In any case, he often shooed me away when Daniela was around. She knew how to make him feel important. She let him carry the shopping basket, push her bike and teach her German, giving her hours of lessons in pronunciation and grammar at a time when he couldn't even name his four children. Asked why he went to such efforts, he said that he was doing it to make sure she wouldn't go.

So at least for one big blonde woman from Nitra in Slovakia, it was a tearful occasion when we decided, in March 2009, that it was time for our father to go, as we say, into a home. Anna had thrown in the towel after her very first three-week stay in his house and, after the past year, any hope that things would improve had disappeared. The days when he refused to cooperate were only increasing. That was the straw that broke the camel's back.

Convention decrees that when you decide it's time for a close member of your family to go into a home, you do so with a bad conscience. And of course such a decision is unsettling. However, there's no harm in questioning conventions. The village's home for the elderly is staffed by trained professionals, working in good conditions. Any problems that arise can be discussed in the team. And they had known our father before he became ill. In the home, they see him as a whole person, someone with a long life, including a childhood and youth, someone who has been August Geiger for more than eighty years and not just since his illness.

In his own home, care at that level was no longer possible, not even with his family's concerted support. Admitting defeat can be a kind of success. Caring for our father was no good if it meant that other family members were neglected. For years everything had revolved around our sick father. Anyone else who had a problem had to deal with it alone. It was stressful enough for us to have our father to worry about day and night. Always the same question: what comes next? We were burdened beyond what we could bear.

On top of all of that, our father no longer felt comfortable in his own house.

His last day in his house began like the other days since his medicine had been changed – without any trace of his former unwillingness to cooperate. Nevertheless, we thought it best to try the home. He got up, dried himself on his own after his shower, and then ate his breakfast slowly and contentedly. It was a warm, sunny morning, so my mother – who had arrived after Anna had quit – took him out to his chair in the garden, where he exchanged a few words with passing neighbours. Meanwhile my mother sewed nametags onto his clothes, even onto his handkerchiefs.

At lunch he ate *Käsknöpfle*, egg noodles in a cheese sauce, then lay down in the living room and nodded off within minutes. He woke up around three, had a cup of tea, and then helped to carry his travel bag to the car. Then he got in and let my mother drive him to the home.

A former councillor sitting by the front door got up and opened it. He seemed to know that the automatic mechanism was broken. My father didn't recognise him and simply greeted him politely.

There was a small woman sitting on a sofa in the lobby. My father waved and exclaimed, 'Hallelujah!' He went over to the woman and took her by the hand. Both of them followed my mother to the door of the common area. The manager greeted my father and showed him the way to his room, where the pictures of his grandparents had already been hung. He said he'd seen those people before but that he didn't know them. The manager had a few more questions about his habits and his medicine, and then she took him out into the garden, where he sat down in the shade with the other residents. It looked like he was happy. After a while, my mother said goodbye. My father lifted his hand and waved.

*

When I walked in a few days later, I found him sitting on his own at his table. I waited a little, then sat down next to him. We talked and arm-wrestled. He pushed for all he was worth, and the wrinkled skin on his face stretched taut in a happy grin. He was obviously really enjoying it. He was not a man forced to live out his life. Though his condition might not have justified his cheerful attitude, it didn't matter. I said, 'You've always been strong.'

He grinned again and replied, 'I'm not strong enough to throw someone into the snow these days, but I'm not peanuts either. I wanted to show you, that's all.'

After a short pause, he added, 'We don't have a choice, in any case, we have to defend ourselves. If we don't, we're no-hopers.'

*

Alzheimer's certainly has not benefited my father, but it has taught his children and grandchildren a thing or two. And the duty of parents is to teach things to their children, after all.

Age, seen as the last stage of life, is a cultural expression that is constantly changing and needs to be learnt and relearnt. And if our father can no longer teach his children anything else, he can teach them what it means to be old and ill. Even this, given the right conditions, is part of a father-child relationship, because you can only take revenge on death in your own lifetime.

Alexandra says her grandfather is adamant he's being mistreated. When Alexandra's mother visits him, she tries to persuade him otherwise. Soon a nurse enters the room and wants to change the nasal cannula connected to his oxygen supply. The nurse says, 'Mr Berlinger, I'm going to push the tube into your nose. It will tickle a little.'

At this, grandfather looks at daughter-in-law, nods vigorously and says, with a mixture of indignation and resignation, 'You see – they tickle me!'

*

Aunt Marianne's grandmother also has dementia. She often says, 'My head is like a churn. I stir and stir, but can't get any butter out of it.'

Aunt Marianne, the eldest of seven children, had to sleep next to her grandmother, until Nana started to say strange things at night. She developed a religious mania. One time, when her priest visited, as soon as he stepped into the room Nana called out, 'I won't have this vile priest in here! Be gone, Satan!'

*

Katharina tells of her grandfather, who also had dementia. When his eldest son biked over for a visit, the grandfather waited for a moment when no one was watching, crept out to the bike, jumped on, and rode away triumphantly.

*

Liliane tells of her mother, who had Alzheimer's. Now and then her mother would look at her and ask, 'Have I died yet?'
  Once, her mother pleaded, 'Please, when I'm dead, tell me.'
  Liliane promised she would. 'Of course, Mum – when you've died, I'll tell you.'

*

Wolfgang tells of his grandmother, who, alive at a ripe old age, had been advised to take health supplements. In the fridge she had a bottle of lecithin. She regularly went to the fridge and, without hesitation, took the bottle of Doornkaat schnapps that stood next to the lecithin. She unscrewed the lid and took a long swig of it, saying, 'Tastes funny today.' Then, just to be sure, she chased it down with a second swig.

*

Norbert tells of a friend whose mother has Alzheimer's. She hasn't recognised her son for a long time. But when the son shows his

mother a picture of himself, she says, 'That's my son!' And yet
she doesn't know the person standing next to her.

*

Wilhelm tells of a friend whose condition had been deteriorating
for years, and yet right until the end he would crawl to his desk
at three in the morning, and, once there, not know what to do.
During the day he would sit there, rolling up playing cards and
trying to light them like cigars.

*

Ursula tells of her great-uncle, August Fischer, who was born in
the same year as my father's mother. In the last years of his life,
Ursula would sometimes pick him up from the home and take
him up the hill to where he used to live. Once, when it was time
to return after a few hours, he asked, 'Do I have to go back to
the camp?'

This great uncle had been a source of fascination in my
childhood. At the end of the lane that passes our upper field,
just before the lane drops steeply to the church square, there
used to be a fountain with an old, half-rotten wooden trough
into which spring water ran constantly. The great uncle, who
remained a bachelor all his life, would bathe in the trough each
morning, summer or winter, firm in his conviction that doing so
would keep him healthy. And indeed, after my grandmother's
death he became the last surviving Wolfurter born in 1898 and
received the remaining monies from the kitty paid into over

the years by and for his year group. As children on the way to nursery and school, we used to watch, fascinated, as he puffed and panted in the water that came, always cold, straight from the woods at Ippach.

*

Christian tells of an old neighbour. She couldn't find the switch for the outside light, so she went out and smashed the light with her walking stick.

And then the illness retracted its claws once again. Our father showed no trace of the tension we had seen over the last few months. He seemed fine to me. He was happy to joke around, play the fool and beam at whomever he was talking to. He was attentive and accommodating.

His impulses were spontaneous. He didn't seem to be in any way 'dimmed' because of his medicine. He had a positive attitude, enjoyed his jokes and gave anyone who would listen good advice. To Werner, he said, 'You can learn from me.'

He had some difficulties with perception, and he did hallucinate, but it was all much tamer than before.

'Did you see the little men, too?' he asked Katharina.

'Yes, they just went around the corner over there.'

And with that the hallucination would pass.

If, exceptionally, the hallucinations proved to be particularly persistent, Eva was called in. She went up to her grandfather, hugged him, and all was right in the world once more. Everyone laughed in astonishment.

My father was still unhappy with what he managed to do. He complained that he was an idiot, but then he'd say, 'I'm not such a complete ass that I can't do anything.'

His weaknesses often reminded him of the past and the 'proud pleasure' he used to experience.

'I used to take real pleasure in the good things I did. I wasn't crazy about all the work, but I knew it was important and that there was scarcely anyone who was as good at those things as I was. Wherever I was, I dealt with everything in a jiffy. Done. It wasn't always lovely work, but it was pleasant. You and I always did well together.'

'I did do well with you.'

'Seriously. We really did. If we hadn't had each other, we would have been shot like dogs. Those weren't things that could just be churned out. Half the things could be, but not everything. I was proud, you know, of those things that only a few people could have made turn out for the best – because *we* could! And they gave me pleasure, because I saw that I could do those things. Things where you needed to work with your brain. I'd tackle them and always succeed. Taking complicated things and giving them the right turn – I was an expert at that. How I managed to twist things this way and that until they were right! And you saw that I enjoyed my work. Everything else would have been hopeless. You all could sense, couldn't you, that I liked the work and that I had a good attitude? I know, there's not much left now. Not much left now at all. I still have some odds and ends, but that's almost the same as nothing. But my achievements back then, all the different things, they were good. I don't know who did it all. I think you were involved. And Emil. And me. I'd get the job done and move straight on to the next one. Just to think, what hard work it was! And when it went well, God, I felt so strong!' He balled his fists and raised them to his chest. 'You know, I didn't particularly think I was an idiot. I knew that when I tried, I'd manage – one time, someone came and praised me because I did it right. He came and praised me. I was proud of how I'd done it. Because, since I used to be pretty intelligent, I could think, *"You've hit the bull's-eye there!"*'

Another time, he said, 'The flukes we had – they weren't by chance. There's always some luck involved, but not all of it is just luck. We were' – he brushed the thumb of his right hand across his fingertips – 'more skilful than the others. So we can't complain.'

*

I certainly wasn't complaining, because I could again look to the future with confidence. All the strain had been blown away. Unusually for me, everything appeared clear – personally, with my family, and at work. We had time to catch our breath. We had landed on our feet again.

Previously, most of my days had ended with dashed hopes, especially during my visits to Wolfurt. At night, my thoughts exerted a dark power over me, so that by morning I was weary, and by midday, as tired as a dog. Even in Vienna, far from Wolfurt, it was not good to let my mind drift homewards. And yet now the days seemed to pass normally again. I was looking forward to the summer weeks in my parents' house. They would compensate for a miserable winter and spring.

My fifth novel had turned out well and for the first time in ages I was light-hearted, something I realised on the day I arrived, when I climbed to the very highest branch of the cherry tree. I hadn't been up there since I had broken three ribs performing a similar circus trick. How liberating to feel joy once more! To wake up and know that I would be able to enjoy the day – that was an elemental change.

The last few years, I hadn't been very adventurous while at Wolfurt. Because some unforeseen incident could occur, I had felt tied to the house. One day after another had passed, sluggishly and yet unpredictably, which is why people in the village saw so little of me. Now, on the other hand, I had not only time but also energy. I called my father's brothers and sisters and his former workmates and told them I wanted to talk to them, for a book I was going to write.

Most of the conversations took place in the evenings. During the day I would pay my father one or two visits.

From the very first day, he was even-tempered, relaxed and attentive. He asked how I was doing and about my plans. He said he was happy enough, but waiting for the right moment to get out of the home.

With a conspirator's air, he said, 'Then you won't see me here any more.'

He leant back and grinned to himself.

He had grown thin. His clothes hung off him. He had a different collar size now, but still wore the same shirts. He was still good with his hands. I found it extraordinarily beautiful that he could do up or undo the top button of his shirt with two fingers, casually, without interrupting his chain of thought. I liked the whole of my father, his entire person. It looked like he was in a good way. I half-remembered a phrase about ending something in beauty. If my father carried on like this, then the same would be true for him as I had once read in a Thomas Hardy novel, which talked of an old man who approached death as a hyperbolic curve approaches a straight line – changing his direction so slowly that, in spite of the nearness, it was unclear that the two would ever meet.

My father's intention was indeed to live a little longer. He was absolutely clear about that.

*

One Tuesday afternoon when I walked into the lounge, my father was sitting with another resident, someone whom he'd asked a few days earlier, 'And who are you?'

'I'm Toni,' the man had said.

At this, my father grinned and replied, 'I think you're more of a *pony*.'

Now, the two of them were deep in conversation. To my joy and amazement I saw that, within the limitations of their illness, they were managing a good conversation, each taking an active interest in the other person.

Toni said he'd been up there, where St Peter lived, and it was beautiful. They all had new flats.

'That's not what I have in mind,' my father replied. 'I much prefer walking around a little and looking for someone to chat with.'

Toni scoffed, 'Well, of course you can't do that up there.'

While Toni and my father chatted, two women were calling for the nurse for help. My father ignored their cries. His cheerful expression didn't change at all, and he didn't even turn his head – he was completely focused on Toni and me. He only paid attention to what was happening behind him when Toni turned towards the women and started to direct withering ripostes at them. He was like the home's own Schopenhauer.

'Help! Help! Won't anyone help me?!'

'Quiet over there!'

'I want to go home!'

'Then call a taxi!'

'I need a doctor!'

'He's gone home already!'

'Doctor!'

'He's at home with his sweetheart!'

'I need help!'

'No one can help you!'

The woman, ashamed, said, 'Oh, I didn't know that . . .'

What surprised me was that although both women were local, their pleas were uttered in High German, as if they wanted to emphasise the seriousness of the situation.

My father was calmly speaking High German with Toni, too, as if they were discussing grave topics.

At a table behind my father, two women were reading the newspaper, undisturbed by the commotion. I found it unsettling that people were crying for help and Toni was just interrupting them. But the staff and residents paid his taunts no more attention than they would a cuckoo popping out of a clock, so I tried to do the same.

But it really grated that, if my father would sing a little, one of the two women reading the newspaper loved to shout, 'Excuse me! Hello! He should be quiet!'

Now my father said to Toni, 'Times are changing, but not for much longer.'

He said it firmly, in a tone somewhere between regret and fatalism.

Toni said, 'I could cross the mountains. I'd like to climb the Alps again. And then head down the Rickatschwende.'

My father replied, 'I won't come.'

'Why not?'

'Because I'm nothing.'

'You're still a lot.'

My father grinned. 'I don't think so.'

'You just have to want it.'

'"Wanting" is not a big thing with me any more. Hope, I do have. In my life, I used to be on my feet a lot.'

Toni said something that I didn't quite catch.

You could see that my father had his doubts about what Toni had said, and he replied, 'Good, I've noted that. What next? The rosary?'

'No!' Toni exclaimed.

'It would take too long.'

'And be pointless. Can you even pray the rosary?'

My father said, 'I think so.'

'OK, so how does it go? Show me!'

My father shook his head and changed the topic.

When the conversation returned to my father's being over the hill and how things couldn't carry on like this for long, Toni said, 'Yes, then they'll put you in a box. Off to the happy hunting grounds with you.'

'I'd rather . . . *chatter* a bit longer,' my father said. 'You know, I can't clear new paths, but I can go here and there, where I can still see things and pick things up.'

Once again, Toni said he'd been up to see St Peter and look around. He liked it up there but St Peter told him that he, Toni, wasn't on the list.

Toni added, 'They've all got new flats up there. You should go.'

My father once again replied, 'That's not what I have in mind. I much prefer to go for walks and look around.'

'You've served out your life already.'

'And you? Do you want to carry on like this for a while longer?'

Toni smiled. 'I'd be happy with a few more years.'

'Yes, you still look strong.' My father undid the top button of his blue, patterned flannel shirt. Then he loosened his tie and explained, smiling, 'I need to let a little air in.'

A thin man in a wheelchair was sitting at the same table. Most of the time he moved his legs slowly, as if he were walking, while his face and torso were quite still. A little taken aback at the sight, my father commented to the man, 'What you're doing there is not particularly effective.'

Toni told my father, 'He spends all day running, at least in his head. In one day, he runs around the whole of Austria.'

'With me, it's the nether regions that are limp,' my father said as he grasped his upper thigh. 'I think it's the nether regions that matter.'

'Your nether regions are still intact,' Toni said.

'I think so.'

'How old are you now, August?'

'Should I know that?'

'Well, yes.'

I helped my father out, saying he would soon be eighty-three. 'Thank you, that's nice of you. I appreciate that.'

'We're not twenty any more, after all.'

'My mother is still fine too. But other than her . . .'

Then, the woman on the couch shouted out, 'Holy sister! Holy sister! Holy sister! Come and help me, please!'

'The nurses aren't such holy sisters any more!' Toni retorted.

Another woman complained, 'I'm so tired! I'm so tired!'

'Then go to bed! Go to your room and sleep!'

'I haven't done anything! Holy God, help me! Holy God!'

'Grant us mercy!' Toni exclaimed.

My father, surprised and happy, asked, 'Really?'

The woman cried, 'Why? Why?'

'Why not!' replied Toni.

To Toni, my father said, 'Even *you'd* pray an "Our Father", if they'd let you work. You still look like you're in fine fettle and would like to work.'

Toni agreed, 'Yes, I'd certainly like to.'

My father added, approvingly, 'You're still strong and solid.'

Toni laughed. 'I've grown solid!'

He told my father that the previous day the paramedics had driven him to the hospital in Feldkirch. He had been itching to tell the driver, a mere kid, 'Out you get – let me drive!'

The two old men talked about making their escape. Then Toni again started to say he'd visited St Peter, who still didn't have him on his list.

'I'd have liked it up there.'

My father said, 'Yes, it can't be bad up there. But I'd prefer to stay in Wolfurt.'

When their meal came and I said goodbye, my father nodded. 'Yes, get home. I've only got one bit of advice for you: stay home and don't leave it!'

*

When I first visited the care home, for an instant I felt pity for all humanity – for those who have lived, for the living, and for those who were still to live. Over time, however, I became accustomed to the unusual situation, and in the end I didn't find their way of life stranger than any other. The constant repetition meant that, on the whole, there was a calm, steady buzz of activity. Even one resident's guttural growls and hoarse shouting, which had annoyed me at first, sounded familiar and pleasant once I knew what a warm nature he had.

My brothers and sister found the home's atmosphere hard to bear. They took our father outside as often as possible. Whenever I asked my sister to tell me about a visit – and she visited him often – she wouldn't want to talk about it. She said that my strategy was to talk about it, while her strategy was to immediately suppress what she experienced there; she was happy to forget everything five minutes after walking out of the door, and the sooner the better. She couldn't find it interesting, just heartbreaking. Reading what I wrote was fine, she said, it even made her chuckle, but the situation itself horrified her.

My younger brother simply said he couldn't deal with it, and he wasn't the only one. Often we brought our father back up the hill to our family home.

Everyone is different, or, as my father would say, 'Our dear Lord has all kinds of lodgers.' Personally, I found the home's atmosphere friendly and enriching, and the staff relaxed and good-natured. They were all local women who used *du*, the friendlier word for 'you' in German, rather than the more formal *Sie*. Most of the residents were full of life – though in a very elemental way. And although the world at large no longer really counted these people among its numbers, they were great company.

*

But then, during my very last visit that summer, my father was not in a good way. A carer from the Philippines greeted me outside the home with the words, 'Oh, thank God, Arno's coming. August has wanted to go home for hours.'

I brought my father outside. He said he was sad about how things were, that he couldn't do anything right, that he wasn't getting anywhere with his efforts to move back into his own house. He hung his head and complained bitterly. Maybe it was because that weekend he'd gone up the hill twice, and just the day before he'd seen his brothers and sisters in his parents' house. Aunt Marianne, Robert's wife, had told me how lovely it had been – everyone happy to see him and no lack of topics for conversation. After all, she said, you don't exactly need to force Paul to tell stories. Apparently, August had listened attentively to Paul and watched him, spellbound, the whole time.

And now, during my evening visit, my father thought I was Paul. He kept asking me what would happen next and whether I could help him get home. His worries had left him drained and he mentioned a number of times how sad he was. I tried to calm him down, telling him we weren't in a hurry and that we could sit for a while longer before we got going. He asked in astonishment, and with a certain shyness, if we were then really going home. I told him we were, we would just wait for Helga and then be on our way. Two or three times he touched my cheek lightly with the back of his hand, and once with his palm, thanking me because my news made him so happy. I had brought a bowl of raspberries and fed them to him, one by one. Later, we went to his room and listened to music. Now and then we would chat. He was still inconsolable, but at least happy he had a brother. After a while, I had the feeling that he had calmed down and wasn't thinking as much about going home. And as it was bedtime and I had to pack for my journey, I stole away. I didn't have the heart to say goodbye. I left without a word and felt rotten. Walking down the hall, I wanted to run back. I thought of the expression 'to tear yourself away.'

That's your workshop. What do you think when you see it?

How much we stored there. I used to think I'd still need it. There are things everywhere with old dates on them. And you, do you work there?

I get a screwdriver or a file out now and then. I like using your tools.

I don't, not any more. I've lost a lot of my mental abilities. If I still had them, I'd enjoy spending time in the workshop.

I enjoy spending time with you.

That's all right, then. I don't feel abandoned or disappointed. I've experienced many things, had many things, achieved many things. It's not so very terrible that only a little more performance is still in me.

I think you underestimate yourself. I don't. You've still got a lot, even if it's not what people normally measure as 'performance'.

Yes, yes, in the past I sometimes did things based on my ideas, but I'm too weak now. Never mind. If I were offended or disappointed, I'd ask if you all could help me. But I'm content enough. I've done a lot in the past. But today – for some time, actually – I don't want to, not any more. For a good while my doing has been going downhill. When I was younger, and grown up, too, I could do a lot. Now, frankly, I can't do anything. No. No. I get it all wrong. But it doesn't make me unhappy that I no longer master things. It's just gone. I can still take pleasure in other people's successes. But I've lost the feathers in my cap.

Our father's house had fulfilled its purpose. It had held together until his children grew up and he had been moved to the home. Now it all looked rather shabby and old-fashioned, and more than one part of it gave cause for concern. Our father had built the house with his own hands. Since the seventies he had been constantly adding to and adapting it. What can I say? Such houses are, indirectly, always self-portraits.

The house gave off a feeling of something makeshift and patched. When it came to his extensions and renovations, our father had normally only asked for help when it was too late. At his day job, he had always possessed the knowledge he needed to work independently. With his home improvements, he'd also had faith in his specialist knowledge – but with less convincing results. Plus, he had developed a near-pathological aversion to throwing anything away. That job was now left to his children.

Our father's eighty-third birthday fell on a weekend. As all of the family was going to be there, our mother had a skip delivered to the house on the Friday. We were going to clear it out.

We got to work and things went smoothly. Everyone felt a load fall from their shoulders as the storage areas emptied and the garden and garage started to look presentable once more. Disappointingly, the skip wasn't nearly big enough for our gargantuan task. After just a few trips it was already full. We hadn't even reached the top floor of the house and there was still stuff piled high in the cellar – stuff he had hoarded for possible later use and yet which over time had become utterly useless. A neighbour, from whom we had borrowed a plastic sheet because it was threatening to rain, had warned us that when they had emptied out their parents' house, they had needed two skips.

By the end of August a second skip was outside the house. My sister had bought our own plastic sheet because rain was forecast again, which was also why we, including Katharina and my mother, got a head start that Friday. On the attic this time. The house is relatively tall: the windows under the gable stand about thirty feet above street level. From one of the windows in Peter's old bedroom, we threw down everything that had been mouldering away in the attic for decades and decades – boards, sheets of plasterboard, boxes of clothes, old bunk beds, doors, chests of drawers, carpets, suitcases, shutters, eiderdowns and mattresses, and some furniture that shattered on impact. There were pieces lying, like a bevy of drunkards, around the front garden.

Among the board games was The Game of Life. Out it went. Done.

*

It rained on Saturday and into Sunday, but by Sunday afternoon the sun was shining, so we got back to work. Our mother fetched our father, and everyone was in good spirits. Our father seemed to be at peace with his world. Walking on the terrace with him, I rested my arm on his shoulder. He gave me a cheeky look and said, 'I see, so *now* you need my help, you lazy bugger.'

'I have to admit, it *is* nice to rest a bit.'

Later, when we were working again, he said, 'I'll help you if you really need me. But I'm stressing the "really"! Anyway, I've said my piece, now you weigh it and see how you'll deal with it. I think you're clever enough.'

At lunchtime he had already told Helga and me how well he'd built the garden fence and how well he'd planned the construction of the house. He was in a bright mood, very eloquent, and enjoying the fact that we were praising him to the skies.

'Yes, we can certainly learn from you!'

And, of course, we did learn something from him: that it's better not to keep everything you could possibly imagine needing one day. What a shocking contrast this attic was to his room in the old people's home! There, he lived in a confined space without the opportunity to store much. And what things does a person need until death?

I often thought about that during the clean-out. For even in the house, there were only a handful of possessions in which my father's life was so deeply inscribed that we absolutely needed to keep them. Most of the things we dragged out were, quite honestly, junk.

On Sunday evening, when it was already getting dark, all four of us children set to work on the cellar – Peter, Helga and Werner in the workshop, and me in the cellar's storeroom. There I found an old coffee mill, a wooden schnitzel mallet, lampshades, the drum from my parents' first washing machine, craft materials, and empty wine boxes. All the dust and mould made me sneeze. I opened the thin horizontal window under the ceiling, just above street level. Peter and I had climbed through this window when he was thirteen and I was ten. We had come home from a snorkelling holiday with a conservation organisation and had been dropped off at one in the morning. I had crept to my bed, where I found Helga, probably because her own bed had been rented out to holidaymakers. As I slipped into bed, she woke up and told me that Uncle Alwin, Maria's husband, had died and was already buried. I had been shocked that things like a burial and an uncle disappearing could happen during my absence.

Such events kept coming to mind now, sleepy echoes that we startled out of their dusty corners.

Helga came out of the workshop with two traps for catching field mice and asked if we still needed them. We didn't, as field mice are practically endangered in

Wolfurt. I remembered how Uncle Paul had replied when I once asked what my father's greatest gift was – 'Catching mice!'

In the spring of 1939, the parish had given a few pennies' reward for every field mouse caught. August and Paul had each earned themselves a bike from their mouse hunting. Paul had only helped out; August was the brains. They had hunted on a neighbour's meadow as well as their own.

Catching mice was seen as a positive thing back then. The parish also gave a small reward for every pound of cockchafers. Josef and Robert took long sticks and a sheet along the Bregenzer Ache river, where there were a lot of broadleaf trees, and in one day they gathered forty kilos of them. For children, this was the only way to get their own money.

*

Swinging my broom back and forth, I swept the dust out the door. By half past nine that evening we were done. We didn't cover the skip this time, because the sky was cloudless and full of stars. I went down into the terrace flat – the very place where I had moved when I was thirteen, thanks to the indecipherable power dynamics in the family at the time. Now the house was quiet. My mother had withdrawn to the top floor, and Katharina had already taken the night train to Vienna the night before. I sat down with my laptop and wrote some notes.

I remembered that Werner had said something that made me prick up my ears. On a little shelf on the wall by the storeroom, he had found various papers, of which some looked very private. He didn't want to investigate any more closely.

I went into the workshop. In a pile of assorted documents, I found a folder with thirteen sheets of paper. On these sheets, at the age of twenty-four, our father had recorded his memories of the end of the war. The folder had lain there for decades and I hadn't known of its existence.

Down the dimly lit passage I stumbled, back to the kitchen, where I sat down with the sheets and read. The war hadn't meant much to him as an eighteen-year-old – it was just a lost year, a topic he dealt with in a few quick sentences. The writing tempo slowed after he left the front. He described in much greater depth his time in the army hospital and his difficult journey home, during which he had been looking for people who spoke his Vorarlberg dialect, so that he could ask for a little bread without it looking too much like begging.

The details shocked me, on the one hand because of how extreme they were, and on the other hand because I suddenly felt that in spite of all my efforts, I knew very little about my father, about where he came from, about his fears and desires.

I had known that while forced to pack up the spoils of war for the Russians, he had gnawed on a rotten bone and fallen ill with dysentery. And sometimes he used to mention that his weight had dropped to around six stone, pointing to the photo he kept safe in his wallet's plastic window. What was new to me was that before the photo was taken, he had spent four weeks bedridden, lying between dying and dead men. Just outside Bratislava, in the hovel that they called an army hospital, they had built twenty-inch-wide racks for the sick. Two people were squeezed onto each rack, forcing them to lie close together on their sides. Given all the infectious diseases and the inadequately treated wounds, it was a death trap.

Unlike the days, the nights were on the cold side, and as the Russian nurses, whom I remember with anything but fondness, only allowed one blanket for every two men, I was sometimes freezing. So I saw myself forced to ask one of my fellow sufferers, one who was no longer bedridden, to try and procure a sweater for me. And in fact the very next morning he handed me one, saying he had pulled it off a dead man in the night, before the Russians saw the man was dead.

For a long time my bunk was right opposite the so-called death camp. It was where doctors sent patients who were so far gone that they'd been written off. These poor people couldn't eat, they bled onto their sick beds, and called out with weak, desperate voices for an orderly when they needed to go to the toilet . . . It was a terrible sight. Almost every day I saw men die, abandoned, with no one to stand by them. Most were fully conscious, but their bodies were just skin and bones.

*

These dead men must have continued to whisper to him in the dark for years. When the dead whisper, they do so stubbornly and insistently. If there were to be a vote on whether it's nicer to be dead or alive, the dead – who are in the majority – would swear it was death.

> *For two days I had a fever, then it broke. It was no sur-prise that I was set to work again, and in fact I had to bury the dead. The ten people who had died in the last few days were thrown onto a hay cart under a few old blankets, after being completely undressed. Eight pris-oners were used like cart horses – through Pressburg's side streets they went, to a scrapyard, where a deep hole had been dug. The dead were thrown in. I had the unpleasant job of filling in the hole afterwards. No one knew how many dead people had been buried in the area. There were certainly a number of graves there already, if you can even call them 'graves'.*

*

My father had never encountered such terrible desolation in the world he came from – people died at home with their families around them and priests at their bedsides. And graves carried the names of the dead. Perhaps that was why for many years on All Souls, my father col-lected for the Austrian Black Cross, a charity that looks after war graves. Apart from that, he never met up with fellow veterans and didn't talk to his children about the collecting. It was something between him and the dead. They inhabited his dreams and his imagination, quietly but powerfully influencing his decisions. That's what the dead do. 'Yes, get home. I've only got one piece of advice for you: stay home and don't leave!'

*

On Sunday night the moon stood directly above the nearest fir tree and shone onto my bed. Towards morning, I half sensed violent winds. They blew newspapers down the stairs to the flat and the rustling paper disturbed my sleep. And yet in the morning the second skip was gone. No one had noticed. We were still asleep when it was fetched. After a brief closing and opening of our eyes the road in front of the house once again stood empty under the sun's morning rays, as if nothing had happened.

Over the next few days, every time we went out in the car my mother and I took more paper, metal and clothes to be recycled. The garage slowly emptied. Only some wood was left, and what we had put aside for the boy scouts' jumble sale. Not much at all compared to what had been there. My mother left again, and I stayed alone in the house for a few days, knowing that my father would never again return to some of its rooms. On Sundays and at family celebrations he would sit in the kitchen and the living room. But his bedroom, now as empty as a dance floor, was no longer part of his world.

I often wandered around the house, moved to think that someone had taken great trouble to create a safe and cosy space here. Now everything had been wrecked – the man, the house, the world. I thought I'd write a book one day with the title *Landscape after Battle*.

It was the time of the third mowing, the beginning of September. Erich, my father's second-youngest brother, was cutting the grass in the orchard with a scythe, all by hand, section by section. I found consolation in his work. Late summer is my favourite time of year. The ruddy apples and yellow pears hang from the tall trees over the mown meadow. There is always a wind that makes the trees sometimes creak like frigates, and children are out playing in the neighbouring gardens. And the shadows of the trees, which have lost so many leaves already, are cast more sharply than ever by the low sun.

From my desk I looked out over the orchard and the nearby houses. Uncle Erich and Aunt Waltraud worked outside almost every day. Once I saw a little Turkish boy who lived in the neighbouring house – he must have been about six years old – run along behind Uncle Erich, who was loading hay onto the cart. I had often seen him 'working' with my uncle. The boy was eating an apple that he had picked up from our orchard and called my uncle 'Grandad', suggesting they were both developing a new cultural identity. The society my father and his siblings grew up in has all but disappeared now. There are still some farming activities, but there's no small-farm way of life. Structural change, as it is called, has turned Wolfurt into a residential and industrial parish. Nowadays, if you plant fruit trees and let them grow to their full height, you receive a subsidy from local government, so that here and there in the village, spots remind people of a culture now nearing its end.

Munching on the apple, the boy bounded across the field behind my uncle and called out a reply to a distant child – 'Cuckoo! Cuckoo!'

He went over to the edge of the field, where two new buildings had been erected on the site of the neighbour's former orchard. The boy watched a young man swinging his daughter around by a hand and foot in their garden before going with her into the new house through its veranda door. The man was the grandson of the woman whose place my father had taken in the care home. The boy ran back to Erich, who was drawing the cart laden with hay back towards his house. Soon the orchard was empty, and the light green stubble shimmered gently.

An airship approached from Friedrichshafen and turned around above the corner of the upper field – as it did several times a day in summer, weather permitting. A buzzard flew over the lower field. Two carrion crows attacked him in flight, stabbing at his back and wings, although the buzzard didn't seem bothered. He certainly didn't attempt to avoid their pecking. He glided leisurely on towards the river.

I thought about how it used to be when there was a storm brewing and fifteen or twenty of us in the family worked feverishly to bring in the hay before the rain. The men shouting loudly in the direction of the tractor that pulled the trailer. The grunt when a forkful of hay was thrown up onto the wagon, where we children grabbed the hay and stamped it into the corners. The quick steps of the women in sandals who gathered up the stalks that had been left. And the steady chugging of the tractor and the rumblings of approaching thunder. And then the mad dash to the barn. On the load of hay, we would lie down flat on our bellies so that the branches of the pear trees didn't clip us around the ears when the tractor drove under them. Little clumps of hay hung from the branches and would remain there for days. And great big rain-drops splashed on our bare legs – legs scratched raw by the hay. And the happy screeching of our younger cousins, who ran along behind the wagon. Someone had gone on ahead, by bike, and opened the big barn door. Accompanied by more shouting, the hay cart was manoeuvred under the overhang. Then the patter of rain on the roof and road. And the air in the barn so hot it was suffocating.

Later we sat in our grandparents' living room, drinking juice and eating ice cream. Then, at home, a shower, our noses full of hay dust, and a quick dinner in front of the television, already too tired to follow the images that seemed part of our coming dreams. Then off to bed, where the raw linen sheets soothed our scratched calves, and immediately asleep.

I also remember that my father and his brothers would meet at dawn to mow the hillside. This would happen three times a year in the late seventies and early eighties. Normally it was five of them: Emil, August, Paul, Robert and Erich. They each brought their own scythe and whetstone. Paul and my father came in their old football boots, because the spikes gave them a good grip, even when they stepped on slugs. The five brothers mowed the steep slope in even strips. The windows of the bedroom I shared with Werner faced the hillside and in the summer they were tilted open, so we would wake at five in the morning at the first sounds of the whetstones. Sometimes two of the men sharpened their blades to the same rhythm, *sh-t*, *sh-t*, while in the background we heard the equally rhythmical swooshing of scythes through the dew-wet grass. That went on for about an hour and a half, and we would nod off as they worked. Then our father and his brothers would shoulder their scythes and head home, before driving off to work in a mortgage bank, in the national bank, in the local government offices, in the forest, and as a meter reader.

As for man, his days are as grass.

A few cuckooflowers here and there.

*

Visiting my father this week, I talked him into arm-wrestling. In the first round, he pulled the wrong way. I explained what we had to do, he understood, and I let him win twice. He had fun, more on account of the 'nonsense' we were getting up to than because he won. He didn't comment on his wins, but said with a smirk, 'People doing what we're doing are hardly needed around here.'

What about old age?

Yes, I get the impression I'm no longer the youngest, that I'm one of 'the elderly' or 'the old people'. I don't give a hoot how people put it.

Are you afraid of dying?

Although it's pretty disgraceful not to know, I honestly couldn't tell you.

It was around quarter to four in the afternoon. Having pumped up my tyres at the bike shop, I rode over to the old people's home. I didn't see my father in the common area, but found him in his room, lying on his bed, his eyes wide open.

He didn't respond when I said hello. I said it again, but his eyes didn't flicker. No reaction at all. I checked to see if he was still breathing. His chest rose and fell, but that didn't stop my heart rate from shooting up. It seemed my voice wasn't reaching him, although I was talking more and more loudly. I thought he must have had a stroke or something like that. But the tenth or eleventh time I said something, he gave a nervous start and looked at me in confusion, as if he couldn't figure out how I had suddenly appeared at his bedside. I asked him, somewhat frantically, how he was. He shrugged and said, 'Good, I hope.'

*

It's said that every story is a rehearsal for death, because every story must arrive at an end. At the same time, by devoting attention to what has gone, storytelling brings back lost things.

Let us sit upon the ground and tell sad stories of the death of kings.

*

Afterwards I sat on a chair and looked out at Lauteracher Strasse, where a car occasionally drove past. Now and then I asked my father if he wanted to go out. He didn't. I tried to make it sound enticing, but couldn't interest him.

'You don't want to go outside with me, Dad? We could go for a little walk.'

'Where to?' he asked.

'Out into the garden.'

'Not interested.'

'To Wolfurt, Dad.'

He looked at me, nodded, and said, as if to prove that he still knew what he loved best, 'Well, that's a different matter, of course.'

He stood up and went to the door. I took his arm, relieved that he was still alive.

*

The further you travel from your origins, the longer you feel you have lived. Were we to measure my father's life in that way, we would say he had a short life until the war, then for a short time he had a long life, and then for a very long time a short life, which only in his dementia once again became long.

*

Another resident in the home shuffled along behind us and asked if the Brothers Grimm fairy tale, 'The Wolf and the Seven Young Goats', could be about infanticide. I replied that he was probably right and that I'd think about it.

As we walked away, my father looked at the man as if he had never seen him before, then promptly forgot him again.

*

My father would say his fellow residents of the home were 'poor fellows, whose willpower shouldn't be measured by their results.' Sometimes he called them 'layabouts' – not excluding himself. He felt good among people like him. 'There are other good-for-nothing layabouts here. I've rounded up quite a crowd.'

Another time he said, with obvious sympathy, 'We've all been patched up.'

*

If I were to compare my father to a literary figure, I would chose Levin, the main male character in *Anna Karenina* – but not just because Leo Tolstoy describes him cutting a meadow with a scythe. What really links the two of them is their wish to improve things. Even today, my father will look around the home's garden and say, 'There are things that could be improved. I can see that with my naked eye. What they've done here looks a bit odd to me. I don't see the point of doing it like this. I don't follow.'

He was often preoccupied with far-reaching plans, declaring, 'I've got plenty of ideas, but they don't come out any more.'

*

I remember how he used to wear baggy trousers and stand under a sunshade to plaster the outer garage walls. Our neighbours, meanwhile, dozed under their sunshade. My father would tie knots in the four corners of a handkerchief and put it on his head, to protect himself from the sun.

*

'And what are they?!'

'They're trees, Dad.'

He raised his eyebrows. 'They don't give the impression of being trees.'

*

Now we sat on a bench in the garden and he was showing great interest in the notes I was making in an old
notebook. He held my book so that it wouldn't slip as
I wrote, and asked me, 'How have you fared with your
papers?'

'I've always fared well with my papers,' I replied.

'Me, too,' he said.

*

It's a strange situation. Everything I give him, he can't
hold onto. Everything he gives me, I hold onto with all
my strength.

*

Such hours seem to go on forever. I have time to notice
so much. Barely anything escapes my attention. I'm lucid,
fully there, everything streams into me so clearly. It's as
if I'm bathed in a strong light.

*

My father kept an eye on me as I wrote, as if he wanted
to say, 'Sit still, son – you have to do your homework!'

*

There's something between the two of us that has led me to open myself more to the world. Which is, of course, the opposite of what people normally say that Alzheimer's does – that it cuts connections. Sometimes it creates them.

*

When our hopes and dreams were dashed, that's when our lives began.

*

Happiness, as death approaches, takes on real weight. Just when we hadn't expected it.

*

To be like General de Gaulle who, when asked how he wished to die, replied, 'Living!'

*

I was barely nineteen when one Saturday afternoon I visited Aunt Berti, Paul's first wife, who wanted to say her goodbyes to her many nephews and nieces. A priest was just leaving the house. She told me that he'd wished her a quick recovery and how ridiculous it was to say that to someone on their deathbed. She looked disappointed and upset. This short moment made a deep impression on me: a dying woman, the mother of three children, two of them still teenagers, demanded in the face of death that no one close their eyes to the facts. I've never quite got over her words.

Sometimes you learn more in a moment than in a whole year at school.

*

That was also the period when we heard the sad news of the suicides of Joe, Maria and Irmi, three of my father's godchildren. It was hard for us to understand those deaths that came out of nowhere, apparently at random, and they haven't stopped weighing on our family since.

When I mentioned them to my father, he didn't remember.

'No, I don't know anything about that,' he said.

On the other hand, his mother, who also died around that time, is now alive again, at least in his mind. 'I have to get home, Mum's waiting for me!'

*

For millennia, *fate* was an elemental force. Today people frown upon talk of fate. Everything has to have an explanation. But at times, things happen to us that we can't prevent or explain. It affects this person and not that one, apparently without rhyme or reason. Why? This remains a mystery.

*

The longing for the years already lived and for the people who have left us behind.

*

One day, my father will draw the breath that isn't followed by another breath. I get angry about all this effort – for what? Then I think there's something in what Julien Green wrote in his diary at the age of eighty: that he didn't mind losing his abilities and dying; God would take the sponge and erase what was written on the slate, in order to once again write His own name on it.

Unlike my father, I'm not very religious. But I can find a secular pleasure in what Julien Green wrote of this Other One writing his name on the slate. Others will frequent places we now frequent. Others will drive down the streets we now drive down. Others will live where my father built a house. Someone will take up the stories I told.

As absurd and sad as this arrangement is, it feels right to me.

*

I read in the newspaper that cockroaches survived atomic tests on the Bikini Atoll and that they will outlive humanity. One more thing that will outlive me. I'm fine with wine and women living longer than me, but that cockroaches will still be here when I've made my exit . . . That stings.

*

Once I was fetching a bottle of wine from the cellar and, as the window by the ceiling was open, I could hear my father talking outside. He sat on the little wall with Daniela and said, 'Maybe the time is coming . . .'

*

If people were immortal, they would think less about things. And if they thought less, life wouldn't be as beautiful.

Without the absurdity of life and the existence of death, neither *The Magic Flute* nor *Romeo and Juliet* would have been written. Why would anyone have bothered?

*

Death is one of the reasons why life appeals so much to me. It forces me to see the world more clearly.

But, to me, since death is an unavoidable reality, indignation about it seems like mere barking at the moon – given how insistently life muscles in.

*

Time will go on, in spite of all protests.

*

I think it's in the film *The Lady from Shanghai* that I heard this little dialogue:
  'I don't want to die.'
  'Me neither. And if I do, then I want to die last.'

*

However much people cling to life, when they believe that someone else's quality of life is inadequate, they suddenly decide death can't come soon enough. That's when relatives start to talk about assisted suicide, though they would be better off considering their own inability to deal with the new situation. Is such talk really about freeing the sick person from the disease, or is it about freeing oneself from a sense of helplessness?

*

Guilty for *still* being alive.

*

I'm never prepared for the moments when my father, with a gentleness I never used to notice in him, puts his hand on my cheek – sometimes his palm, often the back of his hand. Then I realise that I'll never be closer to him than I am in that moment.

*

I'll always remember it. Always. Always! Or at least for as long as I can.

*

I put my arm around him and said, 'Well, you old warhorse?'

'Me?' he asked in surprise.

'Aren't you an old warhorse?'

'That depends what you mean. An old warhorse is strong . . .' He looked closely at me, smiling, and added, 'You're one of those people that always liked a lot of things and absolutely loathed a lot of things, too.'

'Some things I really loved,' I said.

'You always loved adventure. I didn't.'

'What did you love?'

'Going home.'

*

Another time, when I took his hand and squeezed it, he asked me, 'Why are you doing that?'

'Just because,' I said.

He looked at me with a mixture of curiosity and irritation, before replying, 'Of course, you can hold my hand whenever you want. But I do wonder why you're doing it.'

'I'm doing it because I love you,' I said.

The explanation embarrassed him. When he replied, his tone expressed the sense he had that he was no longer good for anything. 'You're just saying that.'

Thrown, I could only mumble, unconvincingly, 'Of course I love you.'

My father's head sank and he dropped the topic.

*

When I ask myself what my father is like, at first he fits easily into a type. Then he once again splinters into the many shapes that he took on over the course of his life, for myself and others.

*

What a bottomless ability to be cheerful he has, to laugh and to strike up friendships.

Coming home from the war, my father's talent for arousing people's sympathy was invaluable. The names of all those who helped him in his time of need are carefully noted in the pages he wrote about his experiences. The ferry across the Danube near St Valentin was paid for by a certain Alfons Mayr from the town of Ried im

Innkreis. Ewald Fischer and Guido Orsinger gave him a loaf of bread in Urfahr. One man forged his Delousing Certificate, so he could hide under the seat of the Red Cross vehicle – a Siegfried Nosko from Dornbirn. One man shared his double ration of food – the music teacher Franz Gruber from Bregenz, who played dance music for the Americans.

*

Almost all of us founder on the ideas we've formed of our fathers. Scarcely any man manages to live up to the image that his children have of him.

*

What could he tell me of the illness, if he were to return from it, like Rip van Winkle coming back from that twenty-year-long bowling night? We would be able to talk to each other differently, more openly, more freely, more intelligently.

It's becoming apparent that in some way his children will come out of these events purged.

*

It is clearly leaving a deep mark on each of us.

*

After many years of living on her own after the separation, his wife has forgiven him for their unhappy marriage. His deep wish for a lifelong relationship finds a kind of fulfilment.

A few days ago, he was back at home, in his house, sitting still on a chair in his kitchen while my mother cut his hair.

*

Particularly in families and couples, you come across feelings that over a lifetime twist around and around, coiling like corkscrews.

*

In the poor man robbed of his senses, I often see my father as he once was. When he smiles at me, clear-eyed, which still happens a lot, thank goodness, I know that my visit was worthwhile for him, too.

It's as if he doesn't know anything but understands everything.

*

Once, when I gave him my hand, he said how sorry he was that it was cold. I told him that I'd just been out in the rain. He held my hand between his two and said, 'Do whatever you need to be doing, but right now, I'm going to warm this hand.'

*

Afterwards we went to sit on the sofa. Once we had decided who would sit where, he said, 'I'm an old boy now. I don't like complicated things.'

Mozart was playing quietly over the speakers. Whenever someone went past, my father would exclaim 'Hallelujah!' and follow the person with his eyes. The fifth time he shouted 'Hallelujah!' the person laughed. My father remarked to Katharina and me with a twinkle in his eye, 'Goes down a treat.'

*

This old man with his small-scale longings that mean more to him than a home in paradise: to go for walks and meet someone with whom he can chat a little.

*

Expectations are modest in the old people's home: little comforts, smiling faces, roaming cats, a joke that works. I like the fact that the people who live here are free from a society that judges people by their performance.

A lack of opportunity is sometimes freeing. In my mind, it's like waiting at a little train station in Siberia, miles from the next village. You sit there and crack sunflower seeds. A train will come sometime. Something will happen sometime. It must.

*

My father took a sip of coffee and put the cup down next to its saucer. He looked at them and said, 'Are they related?'

'Yes, they belong together,' I replied.

'I thought so. Because of their colour,' he said.

*

The newspaper says that black sheep are becoming rarer because of global warming.

*

My fear that the best times are now over has been proven baseless time and again. Whatever I thought I saw coming, it seldom occurred. 'You're way off there,' my father would have said in his level-headed way. So I no longer face the future with such trepidation.

*

Ready for whatever comes.

*

With this book, I wanted to take my time. I saved up for six years. At the same time, I wanted to write it before my father died. I didn't want to tell his story after his death. I wanted to write about a living person. I felt that my father, like everyone else, deserved to have an open-ended destiny.

*

As I write these sentences, I'm almost exactly half his age. It's taken a long time to get here. It's taken a long time to find out something about the fundamental things that have made my father and I the people we are.

*

'I used to be a strong lad,' my father said to Katharina and me. 'Not little kid-goats like you two!'

*

It's said that whoever waits long enough can become king.

Dear readers,

As well as relying on bookshop sales, And Other Stories relies on subscriptions from people like you to tell these other stories – stories that other publishers often consider too risky to take on.

All of our subscribers:

- receive a first-edition copy of each of the books they subscribe to
- are thanked by name at the end of our subscriber-supported books
- receive little extras from us by way of thank you, for example: postcards created by our authors

BECOME A SUBSCRIBER, OR GIVE A SUBSCRIPTION TO A FRIEND

Visit andotherstories.org/subscribe to help make our books happen. You can subscribe to books we're in the process of making. To purchase books we have already published, we urge you to support your local or favourite bookshop and order directly from them – the often unsung heroes of publishing.

OTHER WAYS TO GET INVOLVED

If you'd like to know about upcoming events and reading groups (our foreign language reading groups help us choose books to publish, for example) you can:

- join the mailing list at: andotherstories.org/join-us
- follow us on Twitter: @andothertweets
- join us on Facebook: facebook.com/AndOtherStoriesBooks
- follow our blog: andotherstoriespublishing.tumblr.com

This book was made possible thanks to the support of:

Aaron McEnery · Ada Gokay · Adam Bowman · Adam Butler · Adam Lenson · Agnes Hodges · Aileen-Elizabeth Taylor · Ajay Sharma · Alan Ramsey · Alasdair Thomson · Alastair Gillespie · Alex Martin · Alex Ramsey · Alex Robertson · Ali Smith · Alice Toulmin · Alison Hughes · Alison Layland · Alison MacConnell · Alison N Winston · Allison Graham · Alyse Ceirante · Alyson Coombes · Amanda · Amanda Astley · Amanda Dalton · Amber Da · Amelia Dowe · Amy Rushton · Anderson Tepper · Andrew Kerr-Jarrett · Andrew Lees · Andrew Marston · Andrew McAlpine · Andrew McCallum · Andrew McDougall · Andrew Rego · Angela Creed · Angus Walker · Anna Ball · Anna Glendenning · Anna Milsom · Anna Vinegrad · Anne Carus · Anne Clarke · Anne Williams · Anne Marie Jackson · Annie Allen · Anonymous · Anonymous · Anonymous · Anonymous · Anthony Quinn · Antonia Lloyd-Jones · Antonio de Swift · Antonio Garcia · Antony Pearce · Aoife Boyd · Archie Davies · Asako Serizawa · Asher Norris · Audrey Mash · Barbara Adair · Barbara Devlin · Barbara Mellor · Barbara Robinson · Barry John Fletcher · Barry Magarian ·

Bartolomiej Tyszka · Belinda Farrell · Ben Schofield · Ben Thornton · Benjamin Judge · Bernard Devaney · Bernice Kenniston · Beth Hore · Beth Mcintosh · Bianca Jackson · Bianca Winter · Bill Myers · Bosun Smee · Brenda Sully · Briallen Hopper · Brian Rogers · Brigid Maher · Brigita Ptackova · Bruno Angelucci · Caitriona Lally · Cam Scott · Candida Lacey · Carol Mavor · Carole Hogan · Carolina Pineiro · Caroline Rucker · Caroline West · Cassidy Hughes · Catherine Barton · Catherine Edwards · Catherine Mansfield · Catherine Taylor · Cecily Maude · Charles Bell · Charlie Laing · Charlotte Holtam · Charlotte Middleton · Charlotte Murrie & Stephen Charles · Chia Foon Yeow · China Miéville · Chloe Schwartz · Chris Ball · Chris Gribble · Chris Lintott · Chris McCann · Chris Stevenson · Chris & Kathleen Repper-Day · Christina Moutsou · Christine Luker · Christopher Allen · Ciara Ní Riain · Claire Brooksby · Claire Fuller · Claire Tristram · Claire Williams · Clare Rose · Clarissa Botsford · Clifford Posner · Clive Bellingham · Colin Burrow · Colin Matthews · Colin Tucker · Courtney Lilly · Craig Barney · Dan Pope · Dana Behrman · Daniel Arnold · Daniel Carpenter · Daniel Gillespie · Daniel Hahn ·

Daniel Rice · Daniel T Stewart · Daniela Steierberg · Daria Stokoz · Dario Munoz · Dave Lander · Davi Rocha · David Gould · David Hebblethwaite · David Hedges · David Higgins · David Johnson-Davies · David Johnstone · David Jones · David F Long · David Miller · David Shriver · David Smith · Debbie Kinsey · Denis Stillewagt and Anca Fronescu · Diana Fox Carney · Dominique Brocard · Ed Tallent · Elaine Kennedy · Elaine Rassaby · Eleanor Maier · Elie Howe · Eliza O'Toole · Elizabeth Heighway · Ellen Jones · Emile Bojesen · Emily Diamand · Emily Jeremiah · Emily McLean-Inglis · Emily Taylor · Emily Yaewon Lee & Gregory Limpens · Emma Bielecki · Emma Louise Grove · Emma Perry · Emma Pope · Emmanuel Godin · Eric E Rubeo · Eva Hdoherty · Eva Tobler-Zumstein · Ewan Tant · Felicity Box · Finbarr Farragher · Finnuala Butler · Fiona Graham · Fran Sanderson · Frances Hazelton · Francesca Caracciolo · Francis Taylor · Friederike Knabe · Gabrielle Crockatt · Gale Pryor · Gary Dickson · Gawain Espley · Gemma Tipton · Genevra Richardson · Geoff Thrower · Geoffrey Cohen · Geoffrey Fletcher · Geoffrey Urland · George Wilkinson ·

George Sandison & Daniela Laterza · Gerard Mehigan · Gerry Craddock · Gill Boag-Munroe · Gill Ord · Gillian Grant · Gillian Spencer · Gordon Cameron · Graham R Foster · Graham Mash · Guy Haslam · Hank Pryor · Hans Lazda · Harriet Mossop · Heather Fielding · Helen Brady · Helen Wormald · Helene Walters-Steinberg · Henriette Heise · Henrike Laehnemann · Hugh Gilmore · Ian Barnett · Ian McMillan · Ian Smith · Íde Corley · Ingrid Olsen · Irene Mansfield · Isabella Garment · Isabella Weibrecht · J Collins · Jen Calleja · Jack Brown · Jack McNamara · Jacqueline Lademann · Jacqueline Taylor · Jakob Hammarskjöld · James Clark · James Cubbon · James Kinsley · James Lesniak · James Portlock · James Scudamore · James Tierney · James Wilper · Jamie Mollart · Jamie Walsh · Jan Prichard Cohen · Jane Keeley · Jane Livingstone · Jane Whiteley · Jane Woollard · Janette Ryan · Jarred McGinnis · Jasmine Gideon · Jean-Jacques Regouffre · Jeff Collins · Jen Campbell · Jennifer Bernstein · Jennifer Higgins · Jennifer Hurstfield · Jennifer O'Brien · Jenny Newton · Jenny Nicholls · Jeremy Morton · Jeremy Weinstock · Jerry Simcock · Jess Howard-Armitage · Jethro Soutar · JG Williams · Jillian Jones · Jo Harding · Jo Lateu · Joan Cornish · Joanna Flower ·

Joanna Luloff · Jodie Lewis · Joel Love · Johan Forsell · John Conway · John Gent · John Hodgson · John Kelly · John Royley · John Shaw · John Steigerwald · John Winkelman · Jon Riches · Jon Talbot · Jonathan Ruppin · Jonathan Watkiss · Joseph Camilleri · Joseph Cooney · Joseph Schreiber · Joshua Davis · Joshua McNamara · Judith McLelland · Judyth Emanuel · Julia Ball · Julia Hays · Julian Duplain · Julian Lomas · Julie Gibson · Juliet Swann · Kaarina Hollo · Karin Sehmer · Kate Attwooll · Kate Pullinger · Katharina Herzberger · Katharine Freeman · Katharine Robbins · Katherine El-Salahi · Kathleen Sargeant · Kathryn Edwards · Kathryn Lewis · Katie Brown · Katrina Thomas · Katriona Macpherson · Katy Bircher · Kay Pluke · Keith Walker · Kent McKernan · Kevin Winter · Khairunnisa Ibrahim · Kirsteen Smith · KL Ee · Klara Rešetič · Krystine Phelps · Lana Selby · Lander Hawes · Lara Touitou · Laura Batatota · Laura Clarke · Laura Lea · Laura Renton · Lauren Ellemore · Laurence Laluyaux · Leanne Bass · Leonie Schwab · Leri Price · Lesley Lawn · Lesley Watters · Liliana Lobato · Linda Walz · Lindsay Brammer · Lindsey Ford · Line Langebek Knudsen · Linnea Frank · Liz Ketch · Lizzie Broadbent · Lochlan Bloom · Loretta Platts · Lottie Smith ·

Louise Bongiovanni · Louise Musson · Luc Verstraete · Lucia Rotheray · Lucy Webster · Lydia Bruton-Jones · Lynda Graham · Lynn Martin · M Manfre · Madeline Teevan · Maeve Lambe · Magdalena Choluj · Mahan L Ellison & K Ashley Dickson · Mandy Boles · Mandy Wight · Marcus Joy · Margaret Begg · Marie Donnelly · Marina Castledine · Marina Galanti · Mark Cripps · Mark Waters · Marlene Adkins · Martha Gifford · Martha Nicholson · Martha Stevns · Martin Brampton · Martin Nathan · Martin Vosyka · Martin Whelton · Mary Wang · Matt & Owen Davies · Matthew Armstrong · Matthew H Black · Matthew Francis · Matthew Smith · Matthew Thomas · Matty Ross · Maureen Pritchard · Maurice Maguire · Meaghan Delahunt · Megan Wittling · Meike Schwamborn · Melissa Beck · Melissa Quignon-Finch · Michael Andal · Michael Holtmann · Michael Johnston · Michelle Roberts · Miranda Gold · Monika Olsen · Nan Haberman · Nancy Oakes · Natalie Smith · Nathan Rostron · Neil Griffiths · Neil Pretty · Nicholas Brown · Nick Chapman · Nick James · Nick Sidwell · Nick Nelson & Rachel Eley · Nicola Hart · Nicola Hughes · Nicole Matteini · Nienke Pruiksma · Nikki Sinclair · Nina Alexandersen · Nina Power · Octavia Kingsley ·

Olga Alexandru · Olga Zilberbourg · Olivia Payne · Olivier Pynn · Pat Crowe · Patricia Appleyard · Patrick McGuinness · Patrick Owen · Paul Bailey · Paul M Cray · Paul C Daw · Paul Jones · Paul Munday · Paul Robinson · Paula Edwards · Penelope Hewett Brown · Peter Armstrong · Peter McCambridge · Peter Rowland · Peter Vos · Philip Warren · Phyllis Reeve · Piet Van Bockstal · PRAH Foundation · PRAH Recordings · R & AS Bromley · Rachael Boddy · Rachael MacFarlane · Rachael Williams · Rachel Carter · Rachel Lasserson · Rachel Matheson · Rachel Van Riel · Rachel Watkins · Read MAW Books · Rebecca Braun · Rebecca Carter · Rebecca Moss · Rebecca Roadman · Rebecca Rosenthal · Réjane Collard-Walker · Rhiannon Armstrong · Rhodri Jones · Richard John Davis · Richard Ellis · Richard Gwyn · Richard Priest · Richard Ross · Richard Soundy · RM Foord · Rob Jefferson-Brown · Robert Gillett ·

Robin Cooley · Robin Patterson · Robin Taylor · Robyn McQuaid-O'Dwyer · Ronan Cormacain · Ros Schwartz · Roz Simpson · Rupert Walz · Ruth Parkin · S Italiano · Sabine Griffiths · Sacha Craddock · Sally Baker · Sam Cunningham · Sam Gordon · Sam Ruddock · Samantha Sabbarton-Wright · Samantha Smith · Sandra Hall · Sara C Hancock · Sarah Benson · Sarah Butler · Sarah Lippek · Sarah Pybus · Sarah Salmon · Scott Thorough · Sean Kelly · Sean Malone · Sean McGivern · Seini O'Connor · Sez Kiss · Shannon Knapp · Sheridan Marshall · Shirley Harwood · Simone O'Donovan · Simone Van Dop & Tom Rutter · Sioned Puw Rowlands · SJ Naudé · Sjón · Sonia Overall · Sophia Wickham · ST Dabbagh · Stacy Rodgers · Stefanie May IV · Stephen H Oakey · Stephen Pearsall · Steven & Gitte Evans · Sue & Ed Aldred · Susan Ferguson · Susan Higson · Susi Lind · Susie Roberson ·

Swannee Welsh · Sylvie Zannier-Betts · Tamar Shlaim · Tammi Owens · Tammy Harman · Tammy Watchorn · Tania Hershman · Terry Kurgan · The Mighty Douche Softball Team · The Rookery In the Bookery · Thomas Bell · Thomas Fritz · Thomas JD Gray · Thomas van den Bout · Tim Jackson · Tim Theroux · Timothy Harris · Tina Rotherham-Winqvist · TJ Clark · Tom Bowden · Tom Darby · Tom Franklin · Tom Johnson · Tom Ketteley · Tony Bastow · Torna Russell-Hills · Tracy Bauld · Tracy Lee-Newman · Trevor Lewis · Trevor Wald · Val Challen · Vanessa Jackson · Vanessa Nolan · Vicky Grut · Victoria Adams · Virginia Weir · Visaly Muthusamy · Warren Cohen · Wendy Langridge · Wenna Price · Will Herbert · Will Huxter · Will Nash & Claire Meilkeljohn · William G Dennehy · William Powell · Zoe Taylor · Zoe Thomas · Zoë Brasier

NOW AND AT THE HOUR OF OUR DEATH
SUSANA MOREIRA MARQUES

Translated from the Portuguese by Julia Sanches

A nurse sleeps at the bedside of his dying patients; a wife deceives her husband by never telling him he has cancer; a bedridden man has to be hidden from his demented and amorous eighty-year-old wife. In her poignant and genre-busting debut, Susana Moreira Marques confronts us with our own mortality and inspires us to think about what is important.

Accompanying a palliative care team, Moreira Marques travelled to Trás-os-Montes, a forgotten corner of northern Portugal, a rural area abandoned by the young. Crossing great distances where eagles circle over the roads, she visits villages where rural ways of life are disappearing. She listens to families facing death and gives us their stories in their words as well as through her own meditations.

Brilliantly blending the immediacy of oral history with the sensibility of philosophical reportage, Moreira Marques' book speaks about death in a fresh way.

'Raymond Carver once wrote about loving everything that increases me. This book increased me. It is fearless and luminous and full of grace; it travels to the edge of death and finds life there. Its attention to the particulars of love – between the ones who will go and the ones they will leave – is something close to sublime.'

Leslie Jamison, author of *The Empathy Exams*

'A tender, lyrical and intimate meditation on death and bereavement written with great compassion.'

Gavin Francis, author of *Adventures in Human Being*

'It has the quiet intensity and the transformative power of poetry.'

Iona Heath, author of *Matters of Life and Death: Key Writings*

CROSSING THE SEA
WOLFGANG BAUER

Translated from the German by Sarah Pybus
With photographs by Stanislav Krupař

Award-winning journalist Wolfgang Bauer and photographer Stanislav Krupař were the first undercover reporters to document the journey of Syrian refugees from Egypt to Europe. Posing as English teachers in 2014, they were direct witnesses to the brutality of smuggler gangs, the processes of detainment and deportation, the dangers of sea-crossing on rickety boats, and the final furtive journey through Europe. Combining their own travels with other eyewitness accounts in the first book of reportage of its kind, *Crossing the Sea* brings to life both the systemic problems and the individual faces behind the crisis, and is a passionate appeal for more humanitarian refugee policies.

'An excellent book.'

> Melissa Fleming, Spokesperson and Head of Communications, UNHCR

'It's not just the detail in this book that counts. It's the anger.'

> Robert Fisk, *The Independent*

'Bauer's book . . . exemplifies the best qualities of immersive journalism . . . his brave investigation tells us an important truth about the refugee experience.'

> Daniel Trilling, *Times Literary Supplement*

'Bauer excellently re-creates the predatory, tense world of these shadowy men . . . the people-smugglers.'

> Caroline Moorehead, *New Statesman*

'Wolfgang Bauer is a sophisticated and conscientious reporter, an expert on the Arab Spring and its aftermath, and a brilliant writer.'

> Nell Zink, author of *The Wallcreeper*

'Bursting with humanity and humility.'

> *New Internationalist*

'The refugees' stories and remarkable photos provide a counter-narrative to the popular media rhetoric.'

> *Big Issue North*

ZBINDEN'S PROGRESS
CHRISTOPH SIMON

Translated from the German by Donal McLaughlin

WINNER OF THE BERN LITERATURE PRIZE 2010

Lukas Zbinden leans on the arm of Kâzim as they walk slowly down the stairway towards the door of his old people's home. Step by step, the irrepressible Lukas recounts the life he shared with his wife Emilie and his son. She loved to walk in the countryside; he loved towns and meeting strangers. Different in so many ways, what was the secret of their lifelong love? And why is it now so hard for him to talk to his son?

Gradually we get to know a man with a twinkle in his eye and learn the captivating story of this man, his late wife, their son and the many people he has met along the way. *Zbinden's Progress* is heart-rending, heart-warming and hilarious.

'Zbinden invites comparison with Leo Tolstoy's Ivan Ilych.'
Alexander Starritt, Times Literary Supplement

'A jewel of a novel . . . This book is a little *Odyssey*, a little *Ulysses*; the story of one day's journey, skilfully playing in tandem with another, life-long journey.'
Barbara Trapido

'With its slow pace and winning ways, *Zbinden's Progress* casually sidles up and takes its place alongside a number of remarkable recent works [on] the art of taking a walk.'
Ian Sansom, The Guardian

'A tender, restrained celebration of life's simple pleasures, beautifully translated.'
Lucy Popescu, The Independent

THE ALPHABET OF BIRDS
SJ NAUDÉ

Translated from the Afrikaans by the author

If death comes to a loved one, can we grieve alone? A musician travels the world to see her siblings after their mother's death before returning to her plundered home in Johannesburg; a South African trails his lover through Berlin's party scene looking for an antidote to his successful but boring career. Everyone is facing their greatest loss.

'Cool and intelligent, unsettling and deeply felt, Naudé's voice is something new in South African writing.'

Damon Galgut

'The astonishingly diverse stories in SJ Naudé's remarkable collection *The Alphabet of Birds* count among the best in Afrikaans, built on recurring motifs and elements such as music; departure and travel; fairy tales and myths; illness, dissolution, dying and death; cities; a search for provenance and origins; forgetting and remembering; instinct and reason; that which is said or described versus that which remains unsaid or incapable of description forever; and the places and shapes of love in human relationships.'

André Brink

'Here is the beginning of something extraordinary. Profound, complex, luminously written, and brilliantly orchestrated, SJ Naudé's first collection establishes him indubitably as a writer who will reshape the contours of South African literature in years to come.'

Neel Mukherjee

'Beautifully shaped and often heartbreaking stories . . . At once unsettling and deeply moving, this collection announces the arrival of a writer of great humanity and style.'

Patrick Flanery